I0407150

THE
BIG CHEST BOOK

(Original Version, Restored)

by

BOB HOFFMAN

"The world's leading physical director" - Editor in Chief of Strength
and Health Magazine

Originally published by Strength & Health Publishing Company, 1941

PUBLISHED BY O'Faolain Patriot L L C, Copyright 2012

info@physicalculturebooks.com

ISBN-13: 978-1469995090

ISBN-10: 1469995093

Published in the United States of America

To Order More Copies Visit: PhysicalCultureBooks.com

The information contained in this publication is for historical and educational purposes only and is not designed to and does not provide medical, nutritional, or health advice, diagnosis, or opinion for any health or individual problem. The material presented is not a substitute for medical or other professional health services from a qualified health care provider who is familiar with the unique facts of the individual, and should not be used in place of a visit, call, consultation, or advice of a physician or other healthcare provider. Individuals should always consult a qualified health care provider about any health concern and prior to undertaking any new treatment. The publisher assumes no responsibility and specifically disclaims all liability for any consequence relating directly or indirectly to any action or inaction that a reader takes based on any information contained herein.

Be advised that no one should undertake exercises in the nature of those addressed in this book without prior consultation with a physician. Nor does the publisher make any representations concerning whether any of the exercises or suggestions provided by the trainers or physical fitness specialists featured in this book would be effective or appropriate for the reader's needs or expectations. The publisher expressly disclaims any and all responsibility and/or liabilities that might result from the uninformed or misinformed application of the techniques identified herein as well as for any unsupervised physical fitness training.

Finally, the publisher disclaims any and all liabilities arising from the use of any equipment featured in this book and makes no representations as to the utility, safety, or adequacy of the equipment generally or with respect to any specific purpose.

CONTENTS

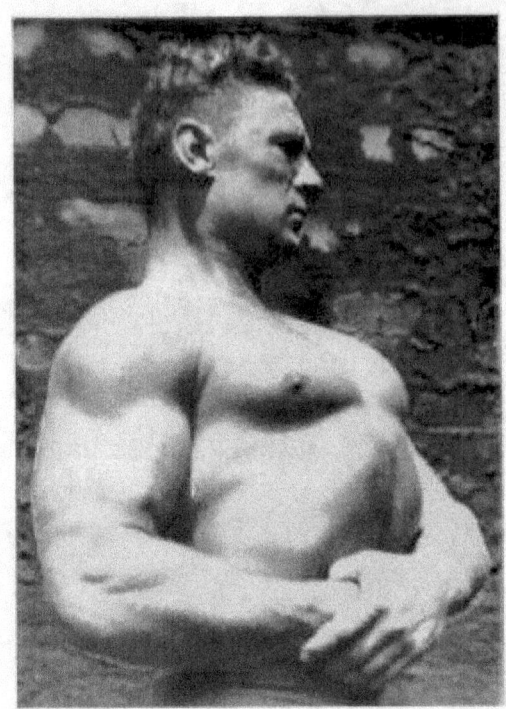

Frank Leight, of the New York City Police, one of the nation's strongest and best proportioned men. He holds the record in the abdominal raise, having succeeded with 130 pounds. Twenty repetitions, ten with each hand, is his record in the alternate dumbbell press with 110 pounds. He was the runner-up in the 1940 Mr. America Contest, won by John Grimek.

Every Man Should Seek a Better Chest

I BELIEVE there is more interest, among those who are seeking physical betterment, in the development of the chest than any other part of the body. Most experienced body builders understand that the building of a larger chest means that the entire physique becomes larger and better developed. Bigger chests mean broader shoulders, more muscles on the outside of the chest, and larger limbs. While less thought is given to the important fact that a larger rib box means more room for the all-important heart and lungs, with an improvement in strength, health, and longevity, this should be the paramount reason for developing the chest.

Regardless of the reason why body builders want bigger chests—whether it is the realization that a bigger chest will mean greater strength, superior health, more vital power and endurance, additional resistance to disease, greater longevity, or whether it is the desire to look better through having a bigger chest—the fact does remain that every man who is seeking greater health, strength and development is interested in building the chest.

I believe that a man with a large, roomy, deep chest excites admiration and commands attention even more universal than the man with broad shoulders or big arms. The vast majority of those who take up the practice of physical exercise do so to look better and to feel better. Although the big, well-developed chest is impressive in appearance and adds to the aspect of the physique when clothed or in athletic costume, the most important feature about big-chested men is the fact that they are always extremely healthy, which of course means that they not only feel well but like the proverbial million.

I have at times written that I am a leading competitor for the title: " World's Healthiest Man." It's impossible to be healthier than I. Few can be so completely free from the slightest pain or physical irregularity of any sort, have such unusual pep and energy, and more than their share of physical strength. I believe that my own good-sized chest has been responsible for much of the wind, endurance and rapid recuperative powers I have always shown in athletics and after enforced periods of heavy work. As you go on reading the chapters of this book you should be impressed with the fact that a big chest provides room for good-sized, powerful, efficiently-operating internal organs of all sorts.

The man with a big chest almost without exception is superhealthy, usually healthy in proportion to the size of his chest. There are exceptions to all rules, but the man with the biggest chest should be, and most often is, healthiest because of the size of his chest; while the man with just big arms or broad shoulders is not necessarily healthy on account of them, but usually is healthy because the exercises which made possible his development have built a big chest and unusual internal strength too.

As we will consider farther on in the chapters on anatomy, the upper chest contains a large part, a highly important part, of the vital organs—the heart and the lungs, in particular; and in the lower part of the chest, the stomach, liver, kidneys and spleen, as well as many important glands. When a man possesses a large, roomy chest box, there is plenty of space for these organs to develop, to increase in size, with a simultaneous increase in internal .strength and vigor.

Some time ago I received a letter which I remember particularly from among the many thousands of other let-ters, for it illustrates how little some medical men know about physical development. Modern, well-informed doc-tors fully realize the beneficial developmental effect, strength of the body inside and out,-which results from weight training. With each passing month more and more doctors become impressed with and " sold " on our form of training. But there still are a few like the one reported in the letter under discussion. The writer of the letter was thirty-six years of age; he told me that he had been interested in weight training for about one year as a result of reading Strength and Health magazine, but before taking up this form of training—using " Iron Pills "—he considered it prudent to consult with his family physician as to the advisability of training with weights. Friend doctor told him not to use weights, that he was too old. He said that weight training would build larger muscles, and as the heart was a muscle it would grow, too; with the enforced breathing which resulted from intensive training, the lungs would strive to get bigger; but a man at his age could not increase the size of his chest as he was too old—past the stage when the skeletal framework could be altered in any manner. With larger organs congestion and serious ills would result.

The man thought things over for a time; he saw the picture of myself illustrating the fact that my chest had grown fourteen inches since I reached a mature age, and he began to believe that he could follow the instructions in the York courses, and probably augment the size of his rib box. He knew, too, that if he felt any sign of congestion in the thorax through the growth of his heart and lungs and failure of the rib box to increase in size, that he could moderate his training, or cease altogether.

He wrote me a letter and asked if I thought he could increase the size of his chest at his present age. I cited my own case of continued growth when past the age of thirty. Most of my chest growth resulted since I found myself in a position to train more regularly ten years ago, when I was thirty-two. A man's nose and ears grow until he is a hundred if he can live that long. The shoulders can be widened and the chest enlarged until the age of fifty at least. Even after that age, there is a good possibility of gaining larger chest measurements by increasing the development of the muscles which cover the chest on all sides.

Bone itself seldom grows after the age of twenty. Some men have grown taller after twenty-one years of age, but they are the exception rather than the rule. There is some broadening of the shoulders through a readjustment of the bones, and a stretching and thickening of the ligaments and attachments which hold the clavicle bones together. The breastbone itself will not grow, but bones of the ribs will spread through the lengthening of the cartilaginous attachments of the rib bones.

I recently received a letter from this same man saying that I was exactly right, for in the first three months of regular training his chest increased in size from thirty-six to forty. In another chapter I will enumerate a few other cases of men who increased the size of their chests to a considerable extent after they had reached an age of maturity.

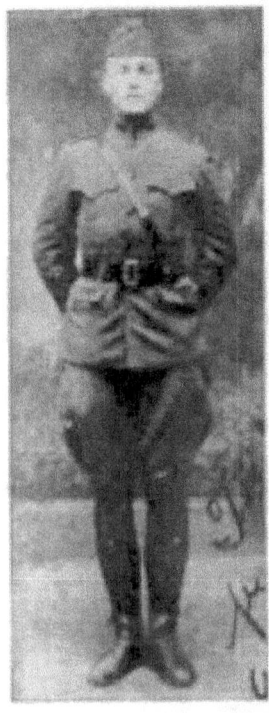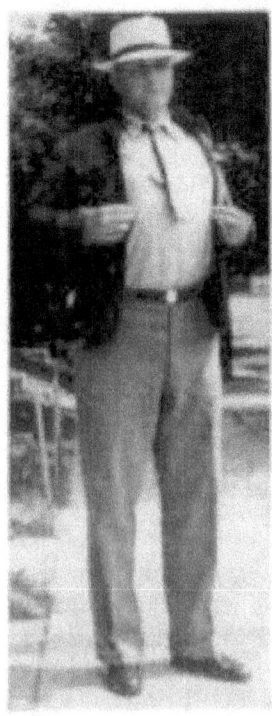

The author in 1919, after the fighting in France, bodyweight 170 pounds, chest 38 inches, and in 1939, weight 265, chest 50 inches. Illustrating his gain of 12 inches in chest size during the years which intervened between the two photos. His chest is now 52 inches, a gain of 16 inches in all.

Nature takes care of her children; if a demand is made upon the body, this demand will be met. If the activities of the body require larger hearts and bigger lungs a greater space will be made for them to occupy. Hundreds of cases are now history, which prove that the chest can be greatly enlarged when well past the age of normal maturity. If a man has a chest of only thirty-six inches, isn't it logical to expect that he also has small organs, and isn't it reasonable to believe that these organs have less chance to cope with various ills and any attack of disease upon their particular selves?

It's a rather homely comparison, but any farmer can look at a group of chicks a week or two old and point out those which will amount to anything. Those that have plenty of chest room and space in the section which corresponds to the lower chest will live and grow and pay their way. The chickens with the longer bodies are the ones which possess the quality of livability and have sufficient resistance to possible disease. Those which remain small and round will probably never grow up, and if they do, they will represent a loss either in weight gained or egg- laying ability. Or ask any man who knows mature chickens and can cull them. Those with smallest chests, with lack of development in the portion of their bodies which holds the organs encased in the lower chest of humans, are the first to be culled; for it is known that they have little chance to continue living—less to lay and pay their way.

A well-developed chest box, which has been greatly enlarged and is in perfect condition, has a much better and surer chance of doing its work well, withstanding any sickness or ills, or to aid in recuperation from any ills which may be contracted due to lack of condition in the remainder of the body.

You are guaranteeing your future health, your strength and longevity by developing your chest. It provides room for the internal organs, strength to protect them, and of course adds to the appearance of its owner. It should interest the body builder to know that the chest is the easiest part of the body to develop, as well as the most important. It can be increased in size more rapidly than any other part. It is not unusual for a gain of from ten to twelve inches to be registered in a year's time by the young man who is going through or has just passed through the period of puberty or of rapid growth. Not so rapid gains are usually registered by men who are older but three to six inches in one year is quite usual. A considerable portion of this growth is the development of a larger rib box, but the muscles of the upper chest, the sides and the upper back account for quite a lot of it.

When a man builds a really well-developed chest, he has little or no expansion because his chest is always near the limit of its possible enlargement. I am often asked how much chest expansion I have, and always .report that I have almost none. If my interrogator apparently doubts this statement I go on to explain that if I would stand in the position of a soldier, with the chest erect, arms hanging naturally at the sides, thumbs along the seam of the trousers, I must get my shoulders back to the point where the chest is held almost at its limit even when not fully inflated with air. Try this yourself. If you already have a good chest, you won't be able to expand much, if any, past the position of attention.

Years ago, one heard a great deal of chest expansion. A man was not considered to be strong and well developed unless there was an expansion of five to ten inches—even more with those who had developed the chest expansion art to the limit. The men who had the greatest chest expansion were never strong men. They were usually men who had performed no exercises except those of a chest expanding nature. If a chest was really covered with firm muscles it could not enlarge to such a great extent. And strange as it may seem, some of the men with greatest chest expansions were those who experienced at least a slightly tubercular condition. The lungs were not so efficient in their operation and thus a much greater area of lung surface was required to perform the normal, moderate work of the breathing apparatus in an inactive person.

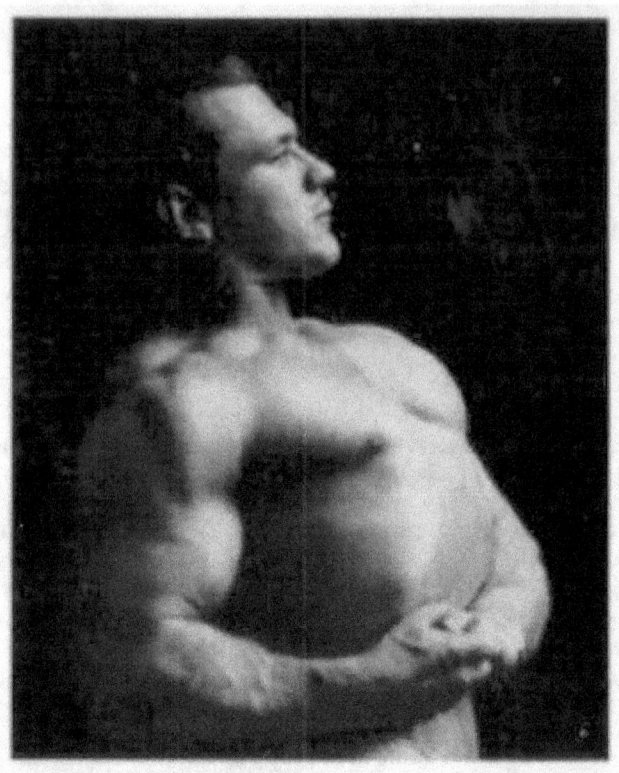

John Grimek, world famous strength and weight lifting star. Among the many honors he has won was his selection as Mr. America at Madison Square Garden, New York City, in the most representative best built man contest ever conducted. He also won titles, "World's best built man," "World's most muscular man," and many others.

A few years ago John Grimek and I went back stage to see a friend of mine who was appearing at the theatre. Another act included a man who was claimed to have the world's greatest chest expansion. From extreme of contraction to maximum expansion he claimed fourteen inches. Contracting his chest, he would place a derby hat under a strap upon the chest. Then removing the hat he would expand until the strap was tight. I told him, although strong men rarely have actual chest expansion, those who are well developed and of good size, having a knowledge of muscle control, can apparently show a great expansion. I said that I believed John Grimek could perform the same feat. Which John proceeded to do, contracting his mighty chest, then expanding it to its limit, with the muscles of the chest, back and sides extended to their limit. You can judge from his photos if you have not seen him in person that this man Grimek has amazing control of his muscles. Off the subject a bit, but another time we were in the side show of Ringling's Circus; a man was displaying his ability there who was billed as " the man without a stomach." He was a man of slender frame, otherwise undeveloped, who had the ability to control his muscles and draw the waist in to an astonishing degree. Although Grimek was so much more heavily muscled, possessing superlative ability at the same sort of feat, muscles and all, his contracted measurement was no greater than the " man without a stomach."

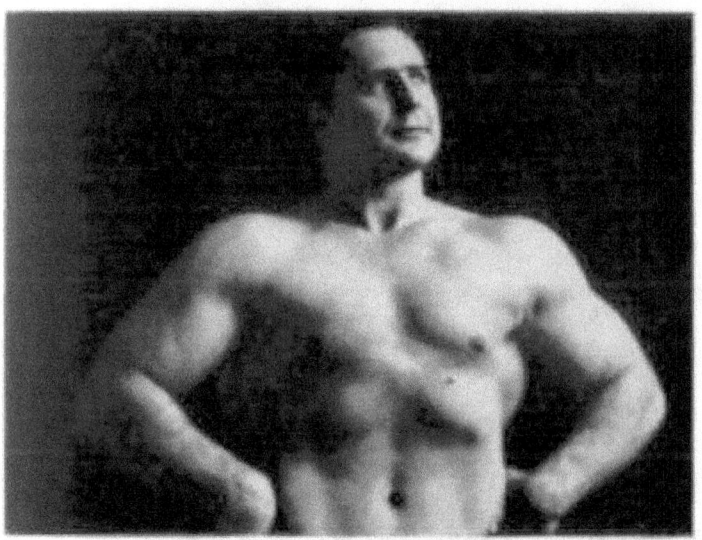

National and world's heavyweight weight lifting champion of 1938, 1939, and 1940, Steve Stanko, of the York Bar Bell Club. Steve weighs 225, has a pair of 18-inch arms and a 50-inch expanded chest.

It has often been said that my friend, Otto Arco, great old time strong man, who is still one of the world's most muscular men, one of the first three men in the world to lift double his bodyweight overhead, has no chest expansion.

In two months of training, the regular training course and a bit of specialization in chest exercises, twenty-four hours of actual training time devoted to the regular, interested and intelligent practice of a few specialized chest- developing exercises, changes in one's chest which are truly astounding will take place. Two months devoted to the development of any other part of the body, the arm, for instance, will bring results, but where the arm might be increased an inch in three months, four inches should be gained in the average case in increasing the chest measurement.

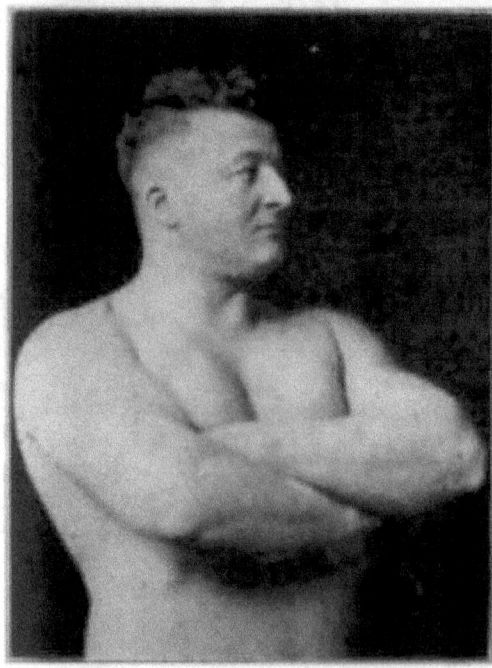

Fr. B. H. B. Lange, C. S. C., formerly director of physical training at Notre Dame University. A well-known and capable writer on bar bell training, he made sensational gains on his own body after the age of 35.

This unusual rate of increase compared to that of any other part of the body comes about, primarily, because most of us—even those with the most sedentary occupations—use our arms and legs to at least some extent. They are better developed in comparison than is the chest. And the chest, being nearly three times as large as the arm in inches of circumference, naturally can gain more in inches to make the same proportionate gain. Three inches in chest gain is no more than one inch gain in arm or thigh.

It's possible to obtain thirty times as much air with resulting oxygen for the body's needs during enforced breathing as compared to the normal respiration of most of us. Even moderate exercise, increasing five or tenfold the operation of the lungs, will create demands which must be met by increased lung size and rib box capacity. Little permanent development of the chest will result merely from deep breathing alone, forcing much more air into the lungs than the body requires. Growth results rapidly when a demand has been made for more lung capacity, and that demand is made by deep breathing with moderate weights to aid the movement. The demands for more air are quickly and permanently met by increased lung size and rib box capacity.

And when the body builder becomes strong enough to work against very heavy resistance, to create an even greater demand for oxygen to meet the needs of the hardworking muscles, then really enforced breathing is necessary and the chest grows by leaps and bounds. The more muscles that are employed in the exercise, the harder and more continuous movement, the more oxygen is required. The deep knee bend is best known as a chest developer, for this movement brings into vigorous play the largest muscles of the body, those of the back as well as the legs, which include nearly half the muscular bulk of the body. Muscles farthest from the heart, powerful enough to vigorously and continuously exert themselves, require great quantities of oxygen to aid the working muscles and of course there is a commensurate gain in chest capacity. Compound exercises of a particularly vigorous nature, such as five movements in succession, each consisting of ten repetitions, exercises which involve all the muscles, such as deep knee bend, dead weight lift, rowing motion with the two hands curl and the two hands press to start the compound exercise, will make such demands that near the end of the fourth or fifth exercise, if substantial poundages have been employed, the body builder should be breathing like he is near the completion of a mile race. When a breathing exercise such as the press on box or some form of the two arm pull over while lying follows such vigorous exertion, greatly increased chest size is sure to result.

Organic Strength Through Developing the Thorax

If you see a man with a big, round, deep chest, what do you think?—that there's a strong, superhealthy man, of course. Public opinion is quite correct in this belief, for a big chest provides more room for the organs which it encases. The lungs and heart have more " living space "—a larger chest box permits them to grow larger and stronger and makes it possible for them to do their work more efficiently.

Few strength and health seekers realize the importance of a large rib box in helping them attain their cherished desire of greater strength and improved health, vigor, endurance, recuperative powers and longer life. Everyone should realize the importance of big, efficient lungs and a strong, enduring heart. The heart starts beating before birth and the lungs commence their lifelong function of breathing an instant after the baby is born. For threescore and ten years, or, as the Bible informs us, "if by reason of strength, for fourscore years," these two organs maintain life within the body.

Briefly, it's the work of the lungs to draw air into the body, extract the oxygen, impregnate the blood with it, which is then pumped or driven to every part of the body. Oxygen is necessary for life. It mixes with the blood fuel which in turn makes possible all bodily movements, pushing, lifting, pulling or carrying. On the return journeys the carbon dioxide is carried by the blood, extracted at the heart and expelled by the lungs. These two organs are partners in most important functions of the body.

Although everyone knows that the lungs are important, they more fully realize the necessity of a strong heart in continuing to be useful and active and to remain in this world longer. When the lungs fail, it is never suddenly. Over a period of many years the little-used lungs will become weaker as a result of less bodily activity. The lungs are capable of extracting the oxygen from an estimated thirty times more air than is needed when completely inactive. As most persons spend their lives with as little physical activity as possible, the greater portion of their lungs is unused. In these deep, dark, moist recesses, germs can congregate, breed by billions and cause consumption or tuberculosis. While there is less tuberculosis today than some years ago, every state has its sanitariums where people with weak lungs must go to spend months to get back to normalcy or perhaps be doomed to spend a lifetime (a shorter than normal life) with lung trouble.

Less thought is given to the lungs than to the heart. When it fails through this gradual weakening process, or this slow insidious creeping of disease, it is less spectacular than the sudden heart stopping suffered by a friend or some other persons—a condition we know as heart failure. The heart will gradually weaken as a result of leading an inactive life; a competent physician's diagnosis may disclose the fact that it is no longer functioning properly. But the majority who die of heart failure are not aware that their hearts are not working normally. Slight pains near the heart are usually attributed to indigestion or muscular aches.

In our own country alone, more than a million people die of heart failure every year, for forty per cent of the total deaths result from a failure of this most important of organs. Hardly a day passes but we read of the sudden passing of some fairly youthful, well-known man. The very young seldom succumb to heart failure, but there is an increasing number who leave our good earth in that manner in their twenties, more in their thirties, with the forties and fifties being the most dangerous time. Heart failure causes men, in particular, to leave this world in their prime, just when they should be enjoying the results of their labors, and with their experience be so much more valuable to the nation through their vocation or profession. When one considers what a man has been able to accomplish in thirty or forty years, before his sudden death, how much more good would he have done in the world if he had lived longer at least the normal span of threescore years and ten. He's taken from the midst of his loving family and is no more.

We must remember that no man can even exist, certainly not become strong and well developed, if he does not have a strong heart. " No man is stronger than his heart" is a good rule to remember. We hear so much of arteries that it's easy enough to forget that the heart is the organ which must propel its life-containing properties to every cell and muscular fibre in the body. You have often heard it said that a man is as old or as young as his arteries. In advanced age arteries frequently stiffen, there is less flexibility, less expansion and smaller quantities of blood pass through them. The heart must work harder, and finally, after year? of battling against these odds, it will give up, perhaps suddenly and spectacularly enough that a man makes the newspaper headlines in a way that he certainly has no wish to make them.

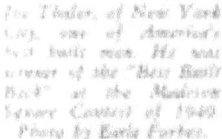

Joe Thaler, of New York City, one of America's best built men. He was winner of the "Best Built Back" at the Madison Square Contest of 1949. Photo by Earle Forbes.

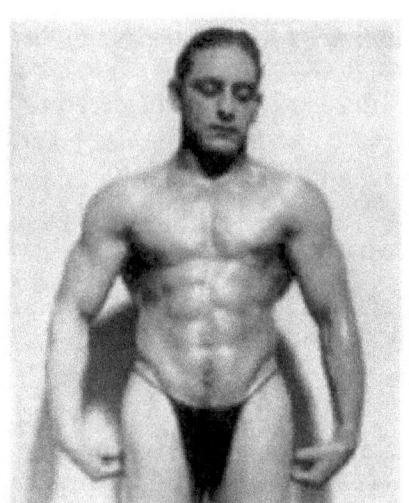

19

You may be saying to yourself, " I know that a lot of people die of heart failure. Uncle so and so went that way and so did grandfather, but what can we do about it? One thing I can't understand is why so many medical doctors, when they find some slight murmur in the heart of a patient, will warn him to cease all physical activity, to take things as easy as possible. He becomes afraid to bend or even to move for fear he'll hurt his heart. The leaders of the American Medical Society, from their learned experience and study of many thousands of cases of heart ailments, inform us that exercise cannot, will not hurt the heart. By this I don't mean that it would be wise to see how far you can swim under water, to see how fast you can run a mile when not in training, or to endeavor to run a twenty-six-mile marathon, play thirty-six holes of golf or a full set of tennis if you are not in training. But the medical authorities as well as leading physical directors do teach that the heart is a muscular pump, a muscle, and like other muscles of the body it responds to exercise and becomes larger and stronger. It's a common belief that athletes commonly die of athletic heart. Of the more than a million persons who die each year of heart ailments, some are certain to have been athletes. A man plays football, baseball, rows or goes out for track during the short years of his college career. Ever afterward he is considered to be an athlete. More than likely when he hangs up his spiked shoes, and concentrates upon making a success of life, he feels that he is too busy to exercise. Like any other muscle, his heart will weaken somewhat through only ordinary use. If the muscles of the arms, legs, or torso are seldom used, never vigorously, they will become smaller, soft, flabby, weak and less enduring.

As the heart is made up of similar muscular fibres it too will weaken with only normal use which is just a fraction of the work of which it is capable. Although it is known by the authorities in the medical and physical training world that the heart is only a muscular pump, that it is not possible to build up enough blood pressure even through the most intensive use to weaken it, there still are many who believe that the heart can be harmed through training.

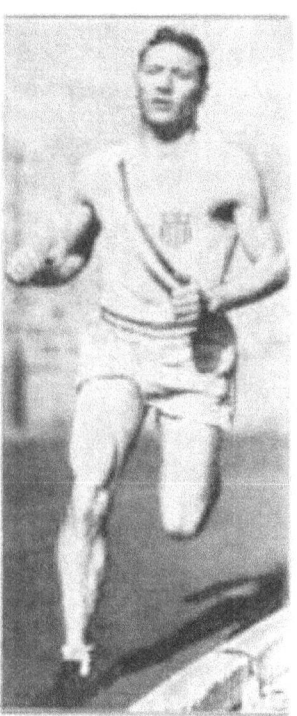

Below: Jules Bacon, of Philadelphia, Pa., one of the newest perfect men. Powerful, he is the possessor of amazing muscular definition and splendid proportions.

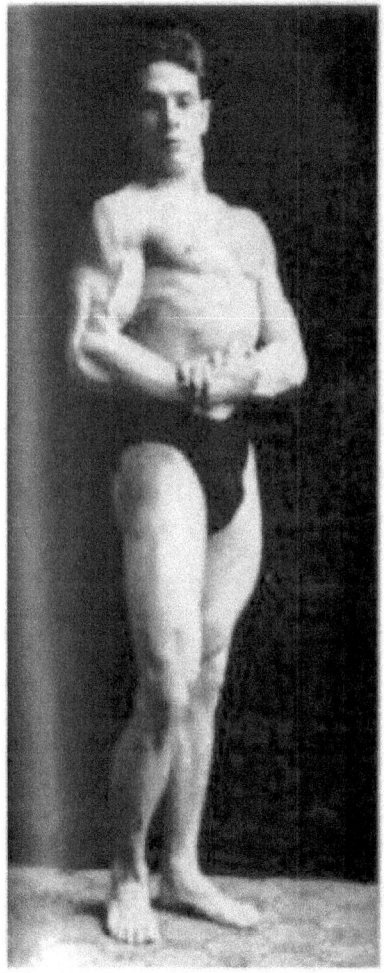

Glen Cunningham, great Kansas miler, member of 1932 and 1936 Olympic teams, many times the annual champion, former holder of the world's mile record. Badly burned as a child in a school fire, told that he would never walk again, with physical training and athletics, he built the sturdy physique pictured here. He has a larger chest and more powerful physique than most milers.

On the contrary, as we will presently relate, it is strengthened through exercise. The former athlete, who has spent long years of inaction physically, still believes that he is " as good as ever," and he is the man whose life is often ended prematurely. In spite of neglect, misuse and abuse of his body he still believes that he is a superman.

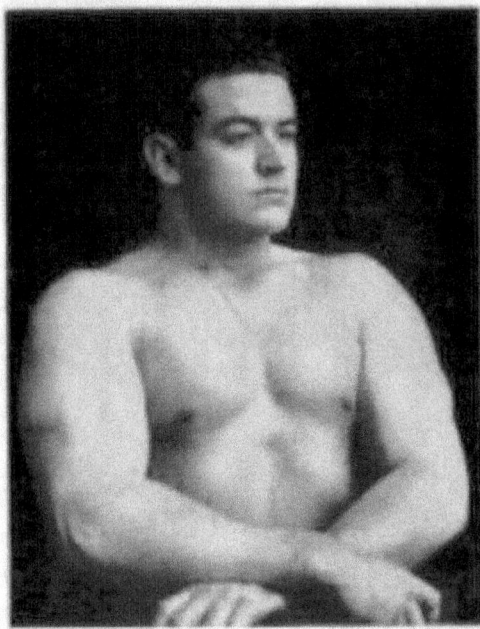

Jake Hitchins, famous York Bar Bell man, who at the age of 20 has already attained a 50-inch chest, an 18-inch arm, and a strong and sturdy body.

I have frequently written that there are two chief reasons for exercise. It makes you look better and feel better. Many men take up the practice of physical training because they wish to build a handsome, admiration-creating figure. There are others, usually the younger fellows, whose sole purpose is to develop the greatest possible strength and the largest muscles which can be obtained. This is a worthy ambition, for since the dawn of history strength has been admired and literally worshipped by men and women alike. Life has always been a survival of the fittest. In this modern day, as in the past, the strongest win the better things of life.

It takes these younger men a while to discover that there is a definite close relationship between strength and super-health. While the very young man doesn't want to read about the organs, anatomy, correct eating or various phases of health—only wishes to learn how to develop his muscles, not realizing that it is not possible to develop strong, good-sized muscles without a knowledge and observance of the rules of correct eating, proper sleeping and the maintenance of a tranquil mind, the average man, usually the older man, will tell you that he doesn't want big muscles. All he wants is health and physical fitness. Like the younger fellow who does not realize that he can't have powerful, well-developed, shapely muscles without observing the laws of health, the man in the opposite category does not understand that he cannot have the health and physical fitness he desires, permanently, unless he has more than average strength.

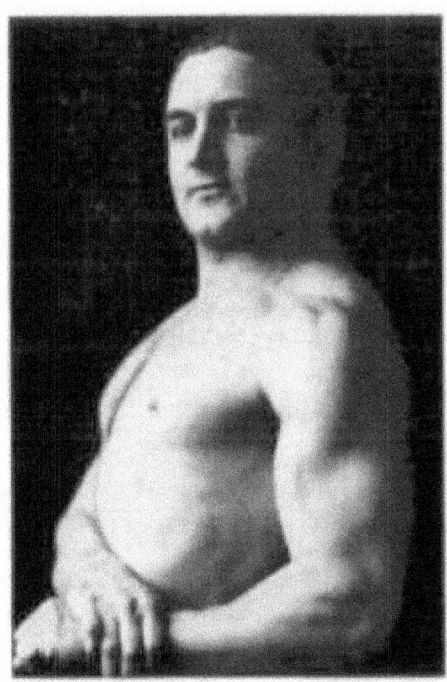

The average man in seeking health, too often, through the apparently easy ways of pills, medicines, and capsules, has not learned that obtaining strength and muscle is the best way to overcome the headaches, indigestion, constipation, colds and many other serious physical irregularities which annoy or even torture him. He may believe that these major and minor ills are a part of life. But the strong men do not experience them, nor do the animals in a wild state. They enjoy perfect health, and possess organs and internal functions which operate with superefficiency.

If every man could realize in how many ways the possession of strength and the health that accompanies it affects our daily lives, even if our work is such that we need not employ strength, they would first investigate the best form of physical training, and then put into practice the proven facts that they have learned.

Older men and women who wish to regain their youthful figures and youthful health and vigor should determine to spend a part of each week in physical activity, for physical activity will improve the action of all internal processes, greatly benefit health, how one feels, and promote longevity. The internal processes and organs are taught to function more efficiently through the demands made upon them by the muscles. Better-operating organs result in the building and storing up of greater reserves of vital energy. Strong internal organs—two of the most important of which are the heart and lungs, encased in the chest or rib box, to the strengthening and developing of which I am dedicating this book—are the result of proper care and exercise.

To live in this good old world of ours longer and more fully you need good kidneys, a capable liver and digestive system and proper elimination. Your future well-being is controlled to a great extent by the capability of your stomach and allied organs, but at the head of the list in importance of your internal works we would find the heart and the lungs. If any of these parts do not perform their work properly, usually a most painful form of illness with ultimate premature death is sure to result.

You depend upon these internal works and they depend upon you. You must take care of them so that they will take care of you. While nearly everyone knows that exercising the muscles will strengthen them they don't know how to go about strengthening the organs. The organs can't use dumbells, bar bells, or cables but they need exercise just the same. You are their partner; it's up to you to strengthen them and to take care of them. Your physical success makes them stronger, more efficient and more successful, and your success, even your life, depends upon how they perform for you.

I believe you are coming to realize the importance of strong, efficient organs. You must believe that they need exercise and you know that they can't take this exercise themselves. Baths, massage and proper feeding are also essentials and it's your task—you who depend upon these organs—to provide the stimulation, the feeding and the exercise they require. Exercising the muscles is the only way to strengthen and beneficially affect the organs.

You must know many men who enjoy perfect health; perhaps you enjoy perfect health yourself at present. I hope you do. If you do, plan now to so organize your life that you will always enjoy more than normal, able-to-be-around health. If you are not quite well at present, plan to so regulate the activities of your life that you will build internal strength and efficiency. If you are one of the men who enjoy perfect health you have a strong heart, big lungs, perfect digestion and elimination; the strong heart and lungs, the perfect digestion, mean that all organs are well supplied with the materials they need to carry on their functions of building, maintenance and repair of all organs and cells. Your mode of living has been responsible for developing these strong internal functions. You not only want to keep them as they are, but plan to strengthen them and lengthen their life and usefulness, for this makes it possible for you to live much longer and more fully.

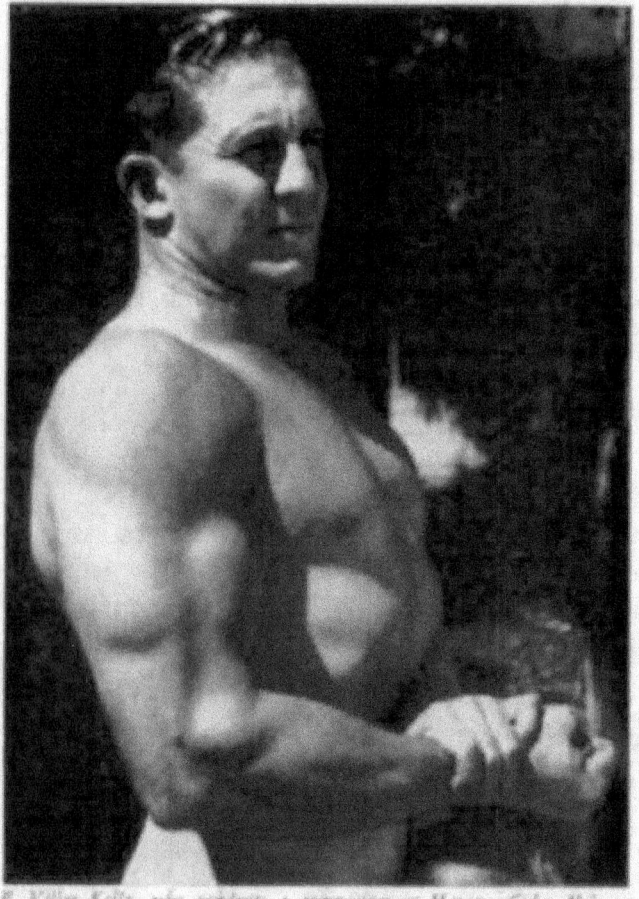

R. Villar Kelly, who conducts a gymnasium at Havana, Cuba. He's an unusually powerful man, particularly famed for his arm and chest development.

You must have observed that the men with perfect health, perfect internal organs, are usually stronger than the average. Think of the strong men you have known. Aren't they supermen; superhealthy too? It's reasonable to believe that there is a close relationship between organic strength and muscular strength. You may wonder, are strong men strong because they have strong organs, or do they have strong organs because they are strong? Strong, sizeable muscles, the result of proper physical training, produce strong internal organs. Similar methods of exercise produce strong, powerful, sizeable, shapely muscles and strong organs. These exercises which build the size and shape of the muscles strengthen the internal organs. It can't be seen but they are strengthened, improved and benefited just the same.

While everyone knows that the voluntary muscles can be strengthened by causing them to exercise or work, few realize that an organic muscle such as the heart can be made more powerful through exercise. The growth and strength of the heart cannot be effected quite as easily as that of a voluntary muscle such as the biceps of the arm, but either the heart or lungs can be rapidly strengthened.

You have often heard the expression, Getting back into training. You know that prize fighters or wrestlers train more intensively before a contest. You know that the members of a football team spend some weeks of training or preliminary conditioning before their season opens. In rowing, if the first race is Decoration Day, May 30th, the ambitious oarsmen have started to work out on the rowing machines sometime in February. Early in March they will take advantage of the first balmy breaths of spring on some fine day to have their first experience on the water. And from then on until the race the crew men will train with ever- increasing severity until they are able to put forth great power over a four mile course and perhaps win the championship of America or the world.

The average man goes out for football after some months of physical inactivity or at least only moderate exertion, unless he is already smart enough to find that he should use graded apparatus such as bar bells, dumbells or cables to not only keep in condition but to better his physical state during the time of the year when he is not actively engaged in his favorite sport. And the football trainer knows that the men in his charge must start out gradually—pass the ball a bit, run a few times around the field, and not participate in more intensive practice for a time, such as " scrimmaging." The preliminary training will wear off any fat which may have accumulated, but most important of all it will improve the action^ of and strengthen the heart and the lungs. A man can be quite strong, but he could not row four miles, run a mile race, or play a full sixty minutes of football unless he has done something particularly to strengthen the heart and the lungs; to improve his wind.

You start out to condition yourself and you run around the track two times. It is hard enough to make these two round trips the first day. But within a week you have increased the distance to four times around and the first two are mere child's play. Each day the work becomes easier, so that before long you can run a mile with strong, steady strides and with only deep breathing as a result of the contirfued activity. The strengthening of your heart and lung action has made this great difference.

In physical training the man with weak muscles and the weak internal organs which accompany them will make his start with moderate resistance and few repetitions. He handles more and more weight as the muscles respond to this gradually progressive resistance. As the muscles are coaxed along, continually trained, as they increase in size, strength and efficiency, their partners, the organs, particularly the heart and lungs, improve likewise. Just as in running, you find yourself able to run a little farther each day, you become able to perform more exercises or handle more weight in the exercises through this bodily conditioning series of physical exercises or activity. You won't see the improvement in your organs as you can see that in the muscles, but it takes place just the same. The added strength and endurance you obtain through various forms of athletics or physical training comes as a result of the work of the internal organs.

The organs provide the fuel for the muscles, feed them and drive them. When you build greater strength and endurance you have actually built better functioning organs and glands. When you run a bit, if you are unaccustomed to it you will soon find your heart pounding and you will be breathing so forcefully that it actually hurts. The lungs will ache and burn afterward. You can feel that the muscular action has made demands upon the organs. The muscles are burning fuel very rapidly, and just as the gasoline in your motor car, or the oil burner in your cellar, requires great quantities of air with its all important oxygen, the working muscles, with the process of combustion which takes place in them, require many times the usual quantity of oxygen. When you become tired, so tired or weak that you must stop, it's because an oxygen debt has piled up. The muscles have been forced to operate without the necessary amount of oxygen. Training makes it possible for the heart and the lungs to provide the working muscles with sufficient of oxygen.

You must have experienced a condition of second wind. It takes place in long distance running. After running a mile or so, depending upon the condition and training of the athlete, he will feel tired, almost exhausted for a time. But after a while as he continues to run he will have more pep, find energy, breathe without distress. A balance has taken place. The lungs and heart have caught up to the demands of the hard-working muscles; the oxygen debt has been overcome and physical activity goes on more smoothly.

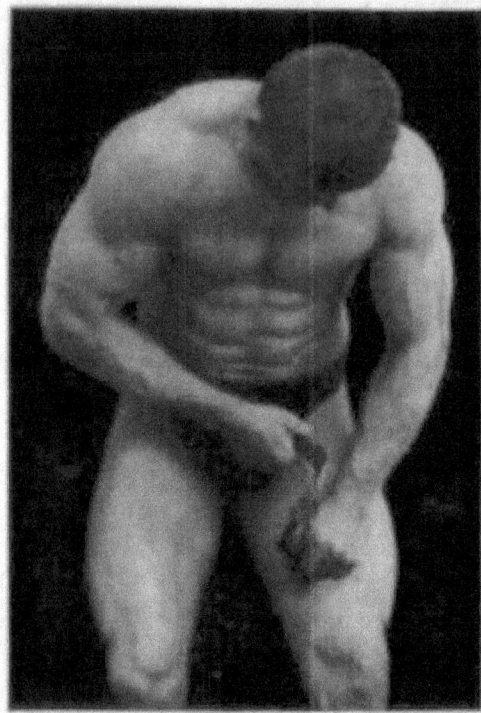

George Hacken-schmidt, "The Russian Lion," where he was world's wrestling and weight lifting champion in 1908.

Training therefore has made possible better operating lungs and heart, and stronger heart and lungs. The special effort amplifies the heart and lung action, breathing is deeper, circulation is improved, worn and broken-down tissue is carried away and it is more rapidly replaced with additional fresh building material. The improved respiration benefits the blood stream, impregnates it with life-giving oxygen which unites with glycogen, providing combustion or power in the muscles. There are other favorable results of exercise which aid the organs in their work. Perspiration, which eliminates much waste from the body, is one of these. The continued exercise creates a rubbing, massaging effect which helps elimination, hastens digestion, improves assimilation. From this you can see that any form of physical activity has a beneficial effect upon the internal organs—chiefly the heart and the lungs. And the more your muscles move, the harder they work, the more work your internal organs have to do. In a later chapter you will read that one of the best chest-developing exercises is the deep-knee bend, and the explanation as to why this vigorous exercise, which brings into action the largest muscles of the body—those farthest from the heart and lungs—is one of the best to develop these important organs. And just as the muscles strengthen with the work progressively demanded of them, the organs strengthen too.

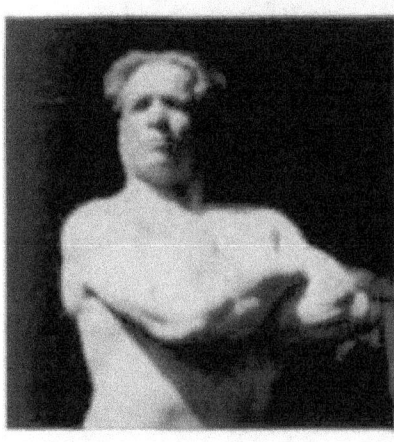

Arthur Dandurand, great old-time strong man, in this recent photo he is 53 years of age. He developed his physique as the ultimate of perfection. Most notable features: 50-inch chest, 32-inch waist, 18½-inch forearm with a 7-inch wrist.

The muscles are trained to run faster, jump farther, lift more weight, and this gradual improvement comes about because the heart and lungs are improving too. The strong-est men have the strongest organs—particularly the strongest heart and lungs. The strongest lungs result from the increased, more intensive breathing. As the heart is a muscle it has been strengthened and generally benefited by the work demanded of it and of course the result of other organic action has caused it to be supplied with the mate-rials it needs to build and strengthen itself.

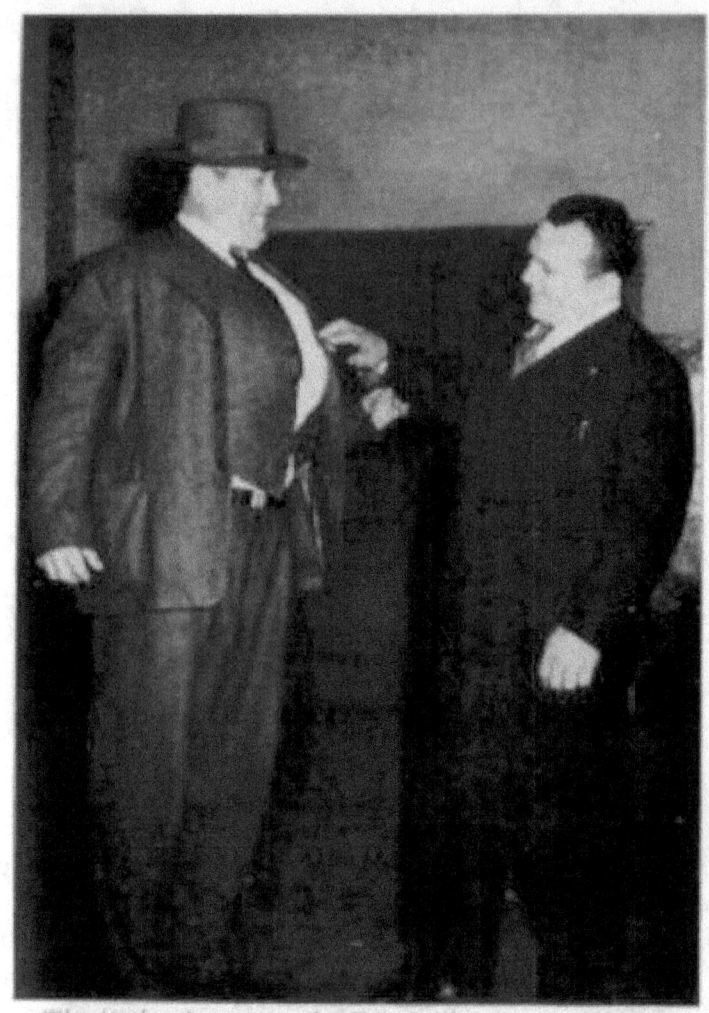

When big-chested men get together. Henry Steinborn, former world weight lifting record holder and champion, for long the strongest man in wrestling, bodyweight 220 pounds, noted for the size and depth of his chest. Bob Hoffman, whose chest was only 38 inches when he first met Henry in 1934, showing what a 52-inch chest looks like.

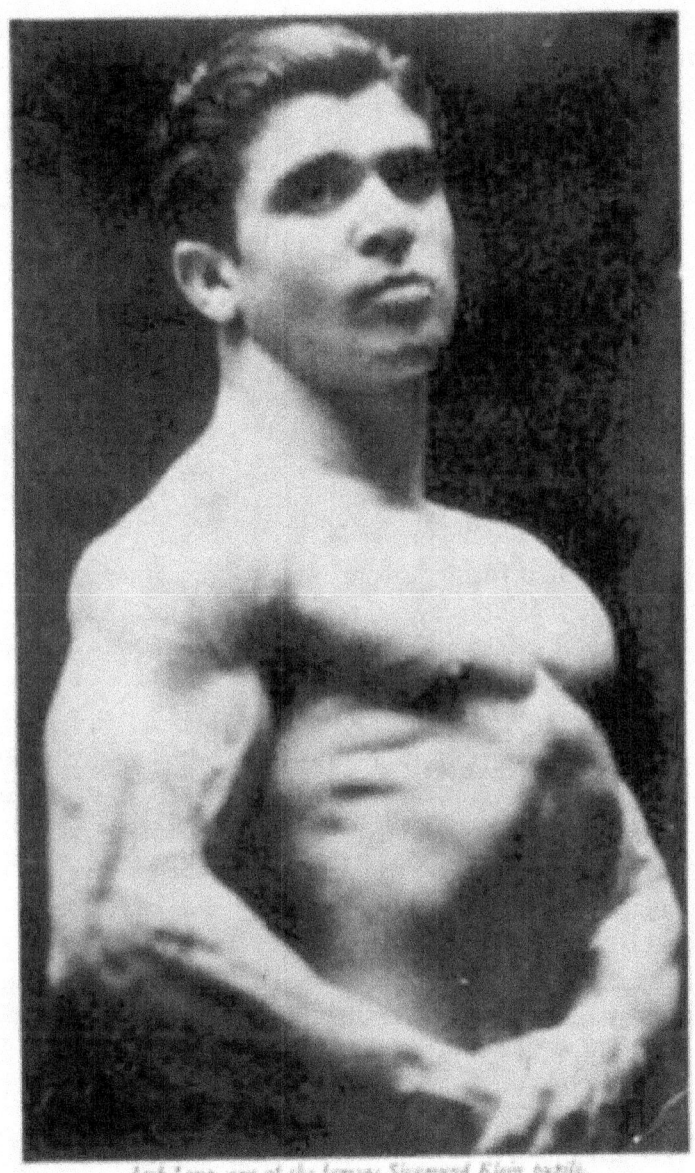

Jack Long, one of the famous Siegmund Klein pupils.

While this book is intended only to supply means for the care and development of the chest, I can't refrain from reiterating once again that this tremendous strengthening of the organs is the reason for the fact that strong men live longer and retain their physical ability to a very advanced age. The pages of Strength and Health magazine have carried the stories of a legion of men well past the threescore and ten age who are splendid physical specimens—far stronger than much younger men who are inactive. It has been told before how John Y. Smith of Boston, at the age of sixty, weighing only one hundred and sixty pounds, outlifted men of larger size and all ages to win the title " Strongest Man in all New England." He's now seventy- five; his friend and training mate, Oscar Mathes, is seventy-seven. There are Warren Lincoln Travis, Prof. Wm. Hermann, Prof. Adolph Rhein, George Hackenschmidt, George Zottman, Joe Lambert, Arthur Dandurand and scores of others who are past sixty, seventy, eighty and even ninety, all former strong men, and so many others— all proof that building strength in the muscles is accompanied by strength in the internal organs. Strong men are strong all over; they have perfect-operating organs; aren't troubled by even minor ills such as indigestion, belching, gas, heartburn, or other minor or major digestive and eliminative complaints; their organs, keeping pace with the increased efficiency of their muscles, synchronize and operate more efficiently when properly treated, which also means properly exercised. All of what I have written is meant to convince you that gradually progressive resistance, gradually increased physical endeavor of any sort, constantly increasing the strength of the muscles so that they can handle more weight, is the road to superorganic action which will in turn result in a longer, fuller and happier life.

As I stated earlier in this chapter, there are some young men who are willing to exercise just for the improved appearance that muscles give them. But the vast majority exercise for the improved feelings which they have learned are the result of exercise. The majority would consider it the height of folly to exercise just to get these muscles on the outside of the body if it were not for the improved appearance, the superior feelings, the happier and longer life the developing of these muscles will produce.

The true facts are that a man must have a perfectly operating heart, powerful lungs, a vigorous digestive system, and a good sound nervous system to enlarge the chest or build muscles on any other part of the body. Modern bar bell and dumbell training, as I teach it, produces the most amazing and beneficial effect on the organs of the body.

Big Chested Men Are Strong and Healthy

Do you remember drawings or statues showing a herculean man who stands with his feet braced, body leaning slightly forward, a huge globe resting upon his shoulders? This figure has been used a great deal in advertisements in recent years to denote the strength or substantiality of the organization which selects this figure as its trademark. I'm referring to the figure of Atlas holding the world upon his shoulders. The story of ancient mythology relates the manner in which the world came to rest upon the shoulders of Atlas. It was originally the work of Hercules to hold up the world; so goes the ancient tale. Atlas should have shared In the labor, but he sought to have Hercules support the world permanently. Hercules, however, had ideas of his own. The story does not tell us that he became fatigued with the work, but it does inform us that he tired of the confining labor, and desired to wander farther about the universe in search of other worlds to conquer. He was reluctant to see others go about their pursuits of pleasure while he had to be constantly at work.

So he did a great deal of thinking. He planned a way to get out from under. He told Atlas that, since he must hold up the world forever, he would appreciate it if he (Atlas) would support it for a short time while he adjusted his lion skin and his pads for the long session of work that he had before him. No doubt this shifting of the world back and forth caused the ancients to believe that there was an earthquake of great severity in some part of their world. Atlas was slow-thinking and it never occurred to him that Hercules might relegate the task of holding up the world to him, when once he got out from under. With his shoulders once more free, Hercules sauntered off, leaving the fuming and indignant Atlas tied down to the laborious and boring task of supporting the entire world upon his shoulders.

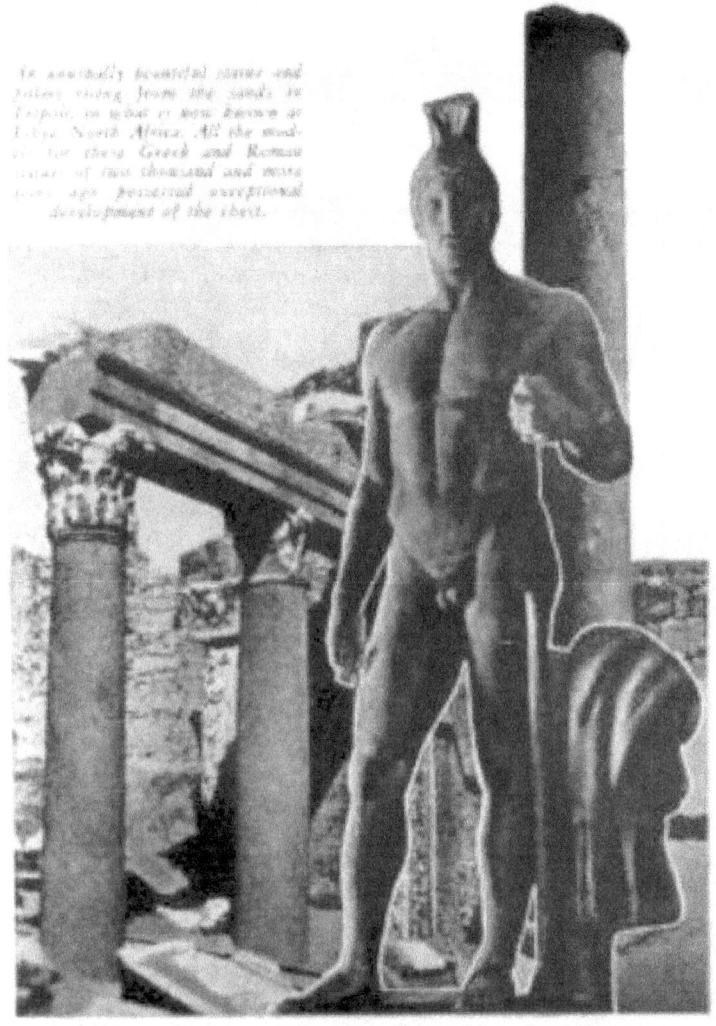

If we are to judge by the paintings and statues the ancient artists have bequeathed us which illustrate the physical development of these two famous gentlemen, Atlas and Hercules, there is little doubt that either of them could carry any burden that was placed upon him. Every ancient statue it has been my pleasure to see emphasized size and depth of chest. There were broad shoulders too, but the size and breadth of chest were especially evident. Throughout the ages it has been known that men with deepest chests are strongest, most enduring, healthiest, and usually live the longest. Few people fully realize the importance of depth of chest.

The rapid development of the chest which is realized by all body builders who launch upon a regular course of heavy, progressive training is most encouraging. The chests of most persons have long existed in inactivity; poor posture has compressed them rather than given this important part of the body an opportunity to grow; the lungs have been compressed and restricted in their action, and when the chest is raised, the shoulders held back, when the almost dormant muscles of the chest region are stirred up and brought into play by proper exercise, an inevitable result follows. Newer and better blood-circulating avenues are opened, the cells are exhilarated and rejuvenated, they are expanded and the muscular tissue increases in size and weight.

There is a great deal to write about the chest. It is one of the most important parts of the body, encasing as it does so many of the vital organs on which our very lives depend. Before going farther I would like to present a question. Do you know just what the chest is? At first thought you may say, " That's a bit ridiculous; why it's right here," tapping the upper part of the chest in the vicinity of the breastbone, the portion covering the lungs. This is not quite the right answer, for it is too general, not sufficiently specific, and to provide a good definition of anything it must be concise and specific.

The chest is that part of the body which covers the lungs, the region under the armpits as well as the part connected with the shoulder blades. The chest is all of these parts harmoniously assembled. By searching for the definition of the word chest in a dictionary we find that the correct answer is a box. And a box, as everyone knows, is composed of four sides, as well as a top and bottom.

Considered anatomically, the human chest is that portion of the body comprising the breastbone and the ribs on the front, the ribs on the two sides and the shoulder blades forming the rear. The backbone is also a very important part of the rib box. All the parts just mentioned form the framework. The framework is covered with muscle, covered with some of the most important (both from the standpoint of health and appearance) muscles of the entire human system. These muscles are woefully weak and neglected in the bodies of the vast majority of human beings. While the limbs of all persons obtain some exercise in going about the daily tasks of living, the muscles of the chest and abdominal regions are too often neglected.

The muscles on the outside of the chest can plainly be seen and are well known to body builders but there are many equally important but little known muscles of the chest which are under the surface. These work in conjunction with the rib box to protect, assist in their function and hold in their place the important organs of the chest region. When the muscles on the outside of the body are neglected, the internal muscles also find themselves in a weakened state after long years of little use. Millions of years ago when every living thing upon this earth travelled on all fours, or at least with the backbone more or less parallel with the ground, the organs were suspended from the spinal column not unlike clothes are hung from a line. Finally some of these animals, which through the process of evolution, so geologists and biologists have informed us, became men, stood up. Then to prevent the organs from piling up on each other just as would the clothes on a line if you held it in a vertical position instead of a horizontal, muscular attachments were developed to hold the organs in their intended place and to assist them in performing their highly important functions.

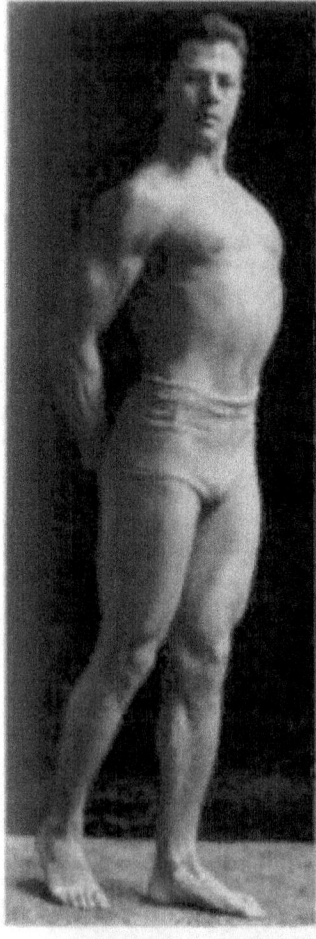

Constantine Kozisis, of Philadelphia, one of the nation's best built tall men. He's a star weight lifter and was winner of the tall man's class in the York Best Built Man Contest.

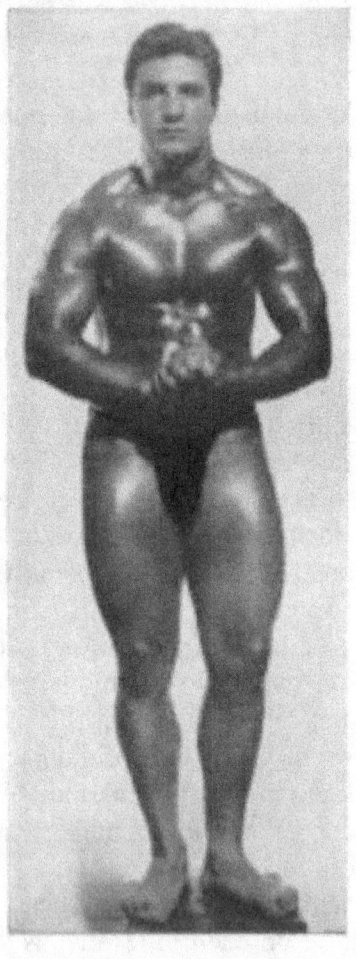

Kimon Vougr, of the Bronx, New York City, age 18, who has been training with weights for three years. His height is 5 ft. 7 in., waist 29, chest 44 expanded, weight 170. Three years ago he weighed 138.

Reasonable exercise, or other forms of at least fairly vigorous physical activity, strengthens these muscles so that they permit the organs to remain in place and function properly. Weakness in the muscles on the outside of the body coincides with weakness of the internal organs. When a person neglects himself completely, many of the organs slip down and add to the protruding abdomens which are a part of so many persons. Fat-incased organs are sluggish, can only partially perform their functions, while those of the man or woman who maintains proper posture and has sufficient internal strength to hold the organs in their proper places enjoy a superior brand of health unknown to most humans.

It must be evident to you who read this that if the muscles controlling, guarding and covering these organs are not healthy, are not strong and vigorous, the organs lying be-neath are very likely to be in a similar condition. And it is just as evident that if the muscles controlling, guarding and covering these various parts of nature's human mechanism are healthy, strong and vigorous, then the various internal parts must likewise be in the same robust, efficient condi-tion.

Therefore the individual who desires to possess real health, superhealth, not just able-to-be-around health, should develop the muscles of the chest, not just one or two—those which can be seen best when exercising in front of the mirror—but all of them, for in so doing he will also develop all the internal organs contained in the chest or rib box.

There are many good chest-developing exercises, scores of which will be offered in chapters to come. The more vigor-ous of these exercises bring best and quickest results. While it's beneficial to walk over to an open window and take a few deep breaths, or to take deep breaths any time of the day you may think of it, it is not to be expected that such deep breathing will create appreciable chest growth. The deep breathing will make you feel better, sort of brush the cobwebs from your brain, for the same blood which serves your big toe and every other part of your body also supplies the brain. All of this blood every few moments passes through the heart and lungs, and the deep breathing will cause the blood stream to be more bountifully impregnated with necessary, vitalizing life-maintaining oxygen, which in turn provides a feeling of exhilaration. Deep breathing is a good thing at any time, for most of us are very shallow breathers, utilizing, while the body is in repose, only about one-thirtieth of the actual capacity of our chests, only a fraction of the amount of air from which the chest can extract the oxygen it requires to keep the muscles working.

It is evident from this brief description and repetition of this all-important physical development truth, which is bound to appear at times owing to its maximum importance, that you cannot expect much if any progress in developing the lungs—thus increasing the size of the rib box—through free hand exercises or just through breathing, without some form of exercise severe enough to demand a great deal more oxygen to continue the greater effort expended. Effort which greatly increases-the body's need for oxygen is required when chest-building progress is made.

Few of us realize how little we use our lungs, how much of the space within the lungs is unused. It remains in idleness as a dark, warm place where cold germs or even more serious disease germs can rapidly multiply because they have ideal conditions for their germination, warmth, moisture and undisturbed quiet. It is good for all of us to breathe deeply at times, draw the fresh air into the lowest depths of the lungs, the innermost cavities, the most remote recesses, filling every tiny cubic millimeter with fresh air. This enforced breathing is a good way to prevent colds.

The divers of the South Sea Islands develop a great depth of chest. It is their work to swim far below the surface of the water to gather the pearl-bearing oysters. The better divers stay under the water for at least three minutes, undergoing considerable exertion every moment they are under the surface. Therefore they must develop great lung capacity to follow their vocations. Unless practiced regularly and from early life, diving and underwater swimming are not a beneficial means of developing the chest, for the continued exertion, with insufficient quantities of oxygen for the body's needs, entails considerable strain upon the heart. When under the water for a considerable period the supply of oxygen is depleted, exertion continues, the heart labors faster and faster and harder and harder, in order to supply the crying need for oxygen. Finally a condition is created similar to the pounding of a motorboat when the propeller shaft breaks or is momentarily out of the water.

Some years ago I enjoyed underwater swimming. I would swim around for an hour or so, coming up for air when necessary and immediately going under again. I entered an underwater swimming contest and, to win, traversed a distance of 123 feet, across a 90 foot pool, and part way back. I continued for 22 strokes after I thought I must come up for air. And my good old heart rattled and thumped alarmingly for many minutes after that exertion.

Great exertion causes unusual effort on the part of the lungs. So much more oxygen is required by the body when it is working hard and long and it is the work of the lungs to extract the needed oxygen from the air and the task of the blood to carry it to the working muscles. There the oxygen unites with glycogen (blood sugar) and forms the combustion or energy which makes it possible for the muscle involved in the .action to continue at the task which has been set for it.

If you were to start out running rapidly, in a short time (or a longer time if you are in training) you would experience a feeling of breathlessness. The breathlessness might result in unusual fatigue, a cramp or pain in the chest. But if you persisted, training with moderation each day, you would find that the parts of the body adjusted themselves in such a manner that you could run without unusual fatigue or discomfort for many miles; that is, if you were training to be a distance runner. This ability to keep going for a long period, to run mile after mile, is what we call endurance. It is accustoming the muscles, but most of all the internal processes—the heart and lungs—to carry on the work they are asked to do, for long periods.

The feeling of breathlessness or fatigue comes about, first, because the blood cannot supply enough oxygen to the working muscle. An oxygen debt piles up; deposits of lactic acid form in the muscles, which cannot be dissipated until the supply of oxygen adjusts itself to the requirements of the body. Fatigue poisons can cause death; in fact they create a condition in the muscles, usually temporarily, like death. The difference is that in life the lungs, heart and other organs are working desperately to normalize the condition they have encountered, and if you are in good condition the internal organs will eventually catch up to the increased output of glycogen and oxygen demanded of them; they will finally be in balance with that of the muscles. Most of you are acquainted with the phenomenon called "second wind." This is renewed energy which comes about when a balance between the output of the internal organs and the output of the muscles is attained. Horses have frequently been driven or ridden at high speed for many miles, to the point of complete exhaustion, the exertion continuing to be so tremendous that there is a greater and greater oxygen debt, no chance for the heart and lungs to catch up, so that poisoning actually takes place and they drop dead.

Most of you have heard of the ancient runner who ran the first Marathon race. The Greeks had met the Persians at the field of Marathon, twenty-six miles from Athens. The actual distance traversed by this ancient soldier ultimately became the regulation Marathon distance. The soldier who made the first Marathon run famous had fought all day, then when the tide turned and his side had won victory, dispersing and pursuing the Persians, he was given the task of running to Athens to notify the worried people of the great victory and the future safety of their country. After fighting all day and running twenty-six miles, he dropped dead just as he shouted, " Victory is ours." He thus gained immortality, but he also proved that the human body or the animal body can be driven to the point of complete exhaustion, or even death, by too long continued unusual exertion. The condition which killed the Greek soldier was an extreme case of fatigue poisoning. Most moderns are so situated that we can stop to rest long before we experience serious ill effects from overexertion.

Eddie Harrison, of the York Bar Bell Club. Overshadowed only by his teammate, Tony Terlazzo, the world's champion, he is a great 148-pound lifter, ranking among the best three or four of his weight in the world.

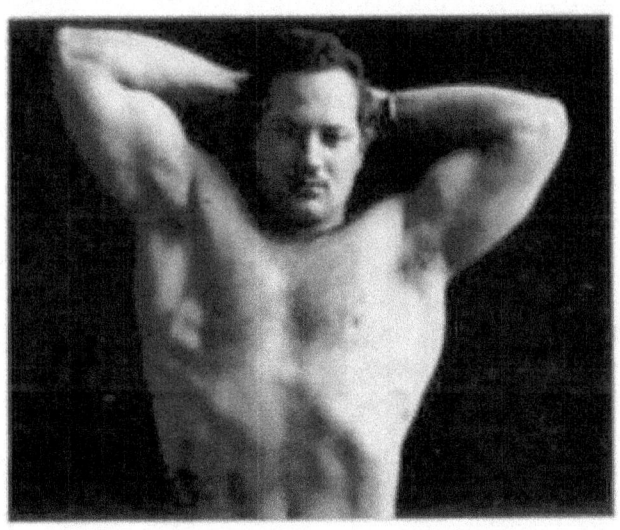

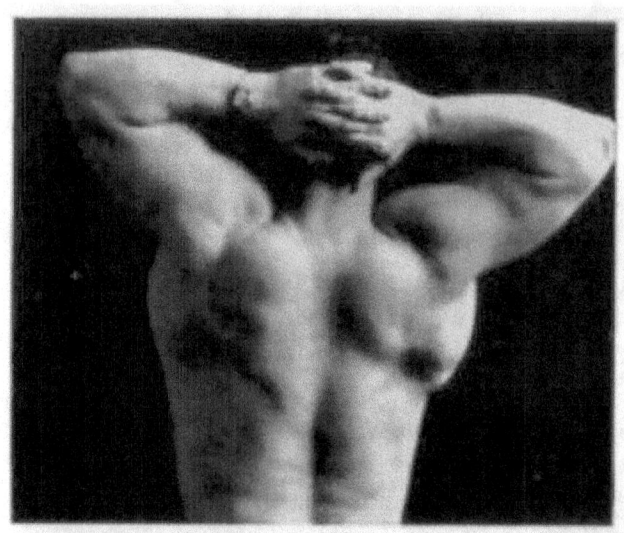

Eddie Harrison again. He weighed 123 and was a star track athlete and swimmer when he first started York Bar Bell training. Fourteen months later he was junior national 148-pound champion of the United States.

To develop a real chest, both powerful and sizeable, real demands must be made. A condition of breathlessness must be created. In our form of physical training this is best attained by practicing any exercise which brings into play or vigorous action all the muscles of the body, particularly the largest muscles, those farthest from the heart, such as the legs. It is impossible to create breathlessness through arm exercises alone. But the legs when exercised vigorously can create an oxygen debt which is manifested by extreme breathlessness. After the exercise which causes the breathlessness, is the best time to practice breathing exercises. In all the York courses, a breathing exercise, some form of pull over with bar bell or dumbells while lying upon the floor, bench or boxes, is listed as the exercise next after some form of leg-developing movement. When you really need oxygen, you can breathe so hard that the ribs will actually separate and you may experience growing pains for some weeks to come. But don't let this worry you; in a moderate length of time you will be rewarded by a larger chest and a much healthier internal condition.

I recently received a letter from a young man who said that he had received his first copy of Strength and Health magazine a short while before. He also sent for and carefully read my booklet, " The Road to Super Strength," which shows a number of before and after cases, great improvement through weight-training methods, and also depicts many of the champions that York methods have built. He said that the book was very well written, whoever wrote it knew his business, but he did not believe he could gain the results in developing his chest that he wanted, through exercise alone. He believed he could get the best results after he exercised so strenuously through swimming or playing vigorous games such as handball, that profuse perspiration was induced and a condition of breathlessness created. And he was sure that he could not do this with exercises alone. That young man should try ten to fifteen repetitions in the deep knee bend with a heavy weight, or even the same number of dead weight lifts with a similar or heavier weight, or practice ten or more dead hang snatches. I consider this latter exercise the best exercise in the entire line of physical training because it brings all the muscles into play, employs all the muscle groups simultaneously and teaches them to coordinate and work in unison. It greatly amplifies or speeds up the action of all internal processes, the organs and the glands which are stimulated by their proximity to the working muscles. It builds athletic ability, skill, speed, timing, nervous energy, endurance and strength. But most of all it induces perspiration, more rapid circulation and very deep breathing. You men who have tried repetition snatching will agree with me.

Chest Improvement Through Proper Posture

WE need power and endurance to put more effort back of our work and the business of living. With power and endurance we can keep on fighting, working and striving for what we hope to win from life. Physical condition is the greatest attribute to success in life, of anything we undertake. The following quotation from the writings of Dr. R. Tait McKenzie should be given thought. He calls for " men " (and of course women too) with clear brains, flushed with blood, driven by a sound heart and purified in capacious lungs, with an unimpaired digestion, erect carriage and elastic step, whose bodies are the keen, well-tempered instrument of the well- trained and well-stored mind. These are the sort of men from whom we can expect audacity in the approach, courage in the attack and tenacity in overcoming those obstacles which stand in the way of success and progress. What a fine interpretation of perfect condition that is!

To acquire a rounded, deep chest and additional strong, well-developed bodily components to go with it, we must take into consideration our position in standing, walking or sitting. Posture is so important in the acquisition of a well-developed, fine-appearing chest and a comparatively slender waistline which improves the chest by the favorable contrast its lesser size creates. A few minutes several times a week spent in chest-enlarging and developing exercises will produce very satisfactory growth in the rib box, providing good posture is made a part of living. If poor posture is assumed for hours each day, it will dissipate the beneficial effects of the chest-developing exercises. Through proper posture, proper holding of the chest, we retain what we have gained as a result of chest-enlarging exercises.

It's customary for most people to permit their bodies to slump, so that an improper curve is permitted on the back.

The head bends forward, nearly resting upon the upper chest. The chest is compressed; the abdomen protrudes. These faulty, careless habits of posture should be corrected in childhood when it is easiest to correct or form any habit. It should be a part of the physical training program in the schools. During youth, before the framework of the body becomes fairly rigid, correct habits of posture should be acquired. While it is more difficult later in life to overcome faulty habits of posture, it can be done.

To improve posture we should start first with the head. The manual of arms, which so many young Americans will be learning since conscription or selective service has become a normal part of American life, and the position of a soldier which it contains, calls for a position of the head so that it is erect, chin drawn in slightly with the axis of the head and neck vertical; shoulders back and falling equally —just how far back will be determined by the next instruction, so that, when the arms are hanging naturally at the sides, the thumbs will be along the seam of the trousers. To assume this position it's necessary to raise the chest and force the shoulders back.

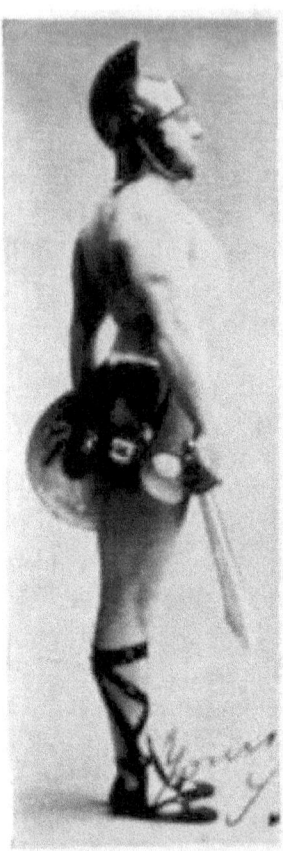

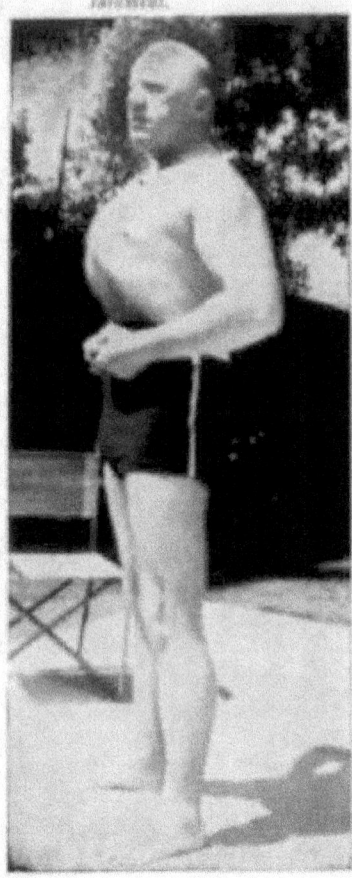

Police officer, Charles H. Thomas, of Burlingame, Calif., weighed 276 pounds. His daughter laughed at him, so he decided to get rid of "old man fat." He weighs 215 in this photo, and need we call your attention to the great difference in waist and chest measurement.

Thomas Inch, of England, formerly England's strongest man.

50

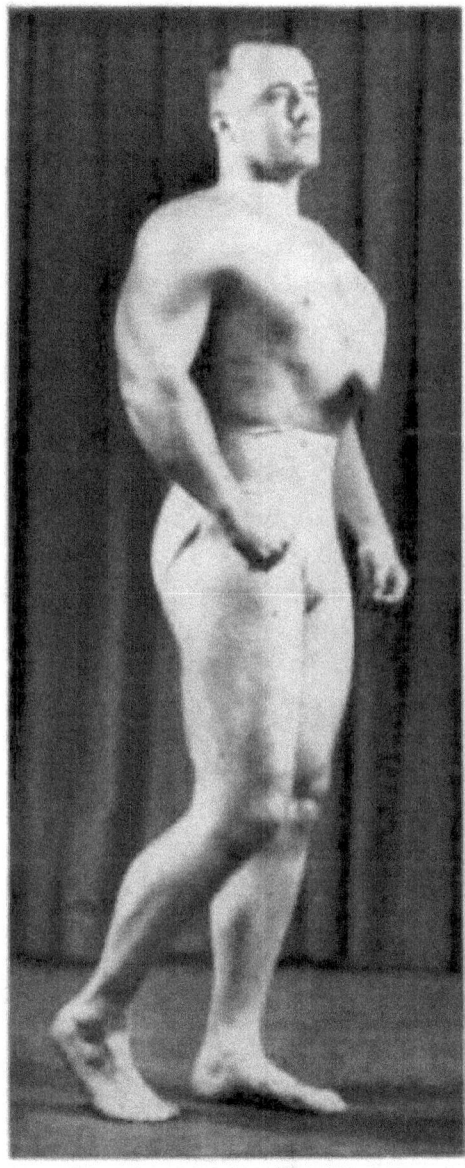

The simple habit of holding the head in the proper position, pulling the chin in, tends to correct the other faulty habits of posture. The back immediately flattens to a more desirable position; the chest rises and becomes fuller. Correcting your posture should take place first in front of a mirror where you can see your normal position and the desired postural changes. It may be a little difficult to overcome habits of faulty posture, which have taken years to acquire, in a few hours or days; it may be tiresome at first to hold the body in the proper position, but the muscles will soon adjust themselves and correct posture will be just as easy to maintain as your former faulty posture.

This year's weight lifting champions—Fiorito, Terry, Terlazzo, Terpak, Davis and Stanko, with the addition of that greatest of all physical specimens, John Grimek—are all examples of good posture. Their good posture has had a tremendous influence on the development of their matchless strength, in their body weight divisions, and their splendid physiques. John Grimek in particular is noted for the great depth, roundness and size of his chest. Coupled with it is a well-muscled but slender waist which is so much smaller than his chest that it seems to be wasplike in comparison. Good posture more than any other one thing has accounted for this splendid development of the chest and favorable contrast in size between the waist and chest. Grimek has good posture at all times. While sitting at the table, or driving in his car, chest is erect, waist drawn in; when standing in the gym his posture is always good. He early recognized the vital need for good posture, and a large share of the physical glory that he has won has resulted from these habits of proper posture which he early acquired.

Your own feelings and the impression you create upon others are determined greatly by the development and carriage of your body. If you slouch, permitting your back to round, your chest to flatten, your abdomen to protrude, you more than likely will experience a lazy, lackadaisical feeling. But if you will contract habits of proper posture, what a difference! You exercise only for an hour or two,

two to four times a week, when you follow a system of progressive training with apparatus, to develop all the parts of the body, but you must always be watching your posture; and particularly if you have spent long years in faulty positions, you should acquire habits of good posture.

Your task is to train your muscles to hold your bony framework in the proper and most beneficial positions. During the day, at your work, whether it requires that you stand or sit at a desk, going to and from work, practice good posture in every position and in every act you must perform.

We exercise primarily for two reasons: to feel better and to look better; and correct posture plays an important part both in how we feel as well as how we look. We form our first impression of a man, of his strength and ability, by looking at him. If he carries his chest high, has depth of chest, with shoulders that are square and held well back, we are duly impressed with the fact that here is a vital man, capable of carrying through any task which may be given to him. But when ye see a man who slumps and slouches along we expect him to have other faulty and careless habits. We feel that he is the type who has a cigarette constantly drooping from the corner of his mouth and spends a good share of his spare time at habits which are not beneficial, to say the least.

Your personal appearance, which is an important part of the whole we know as your personality, weighs tremendously toward your success in life and the happiness you obtain from that life. A well-developed physique, and good posture to show this physique to its best advantage, is a great factor not only in producing a pleasing personality, but the good appearance development and posture engendered is a great asset to any man or woman in any trade, profession or vocation he or she may follow, as well as in all social contacts.

While favorable first impressions are very important, from our own standpoint how we feel is most important. Here a deep, well-rounded, roomy chest is highly important in the promotion of health, vigor and vitality. The chest is the box which contains very important organs on which our well being and very lives depend, and how we carry it and how we build it depend upon whether it will be a little weak box, a middle-sized box, or a big powerful box. In it are contained our most valuable possessions—not gold, silver or jewels, not money or bonds, for all of these are useless to us if our hearts and lungs do not continue to perform their functions. The organs on which our very breath of life depends must be given ample space in which to work; they should not be crowded or they cannot work properly, efficiently and for seventy or eighty years which should be our normal span of life.

If the heart and lungs are cramped, impeded in their work, many ills from which mankind suffers will be present sooner or later. The flat-chested, stoop-shouldered man or woman is far more likely to have lung disorders or even the common colds and catarrh. But give these organs plenty of space, exercise them, revitalize them through creating demands and meeting these demands with ample supplies of fresh oxygen, rich air, and plenty of space in which to work and you will be rewarded with abundant vitality and perfect synchronization of all the organs of the chest region.

All armies of the world and every military academy have placed particular emphasis upon proper posture. It does add to the appearance of a group of men to have them uniformly present attractive physiques on which the marks of good posture are indelibly stamped, but the chief reason for the army's good posture is the knowledge that correct posture and better bodies encourage men, inspire them, give them confidence, make them more enduring, better disciplined, and more courageous. We in civilian life don't have anyone like the drill sergeants in the army to constantly pound into us—inculcate into our very being—the necessity for correct posture; we must be intelligent enough to recognize the need for proper posture, and to constantly maintain our bodies in the most favorable position.

Look around you in any group and observe the poor body mechanics of most of the individuals within your sight. If these people only realized that good posture is an inherent part of good health, and that physical debility and internal disorders are just as surely the result of faulty posture! With less than half of the population of our nation possessing even fair posture, it's not much wonder that we are the sickest nation in the world; that two million of us are constantly sick and unable to work; and that a great many others experience just-able-to-be-around health and strength.

A physical examination at Harvard University disclosed the fact that eighty per cent of the freshman class ranked in C class concerning posture. And many of them were still lower—in the D class. Poor posture is often the result of bodily weakness. Therefore strong bodies should mean good posture. But it is surprising how many well-built fellows still maintain a poor posture. So often an excellent musculature is hardly visible due to faulty posture. You should contract the habit of being chesty. Don't mind if someone kiddingly remarks about your outthrust chest. On one of the trips to the Olympics a member of the team asked me why I was standing with my chest out. I replied that that was the only natural way to stand. If a chest of my size was not out, it would slump and my abdomen protrude. But the man who remarks perhaps disparagingly because you stand or walk with your chest out secretly admires you for it.

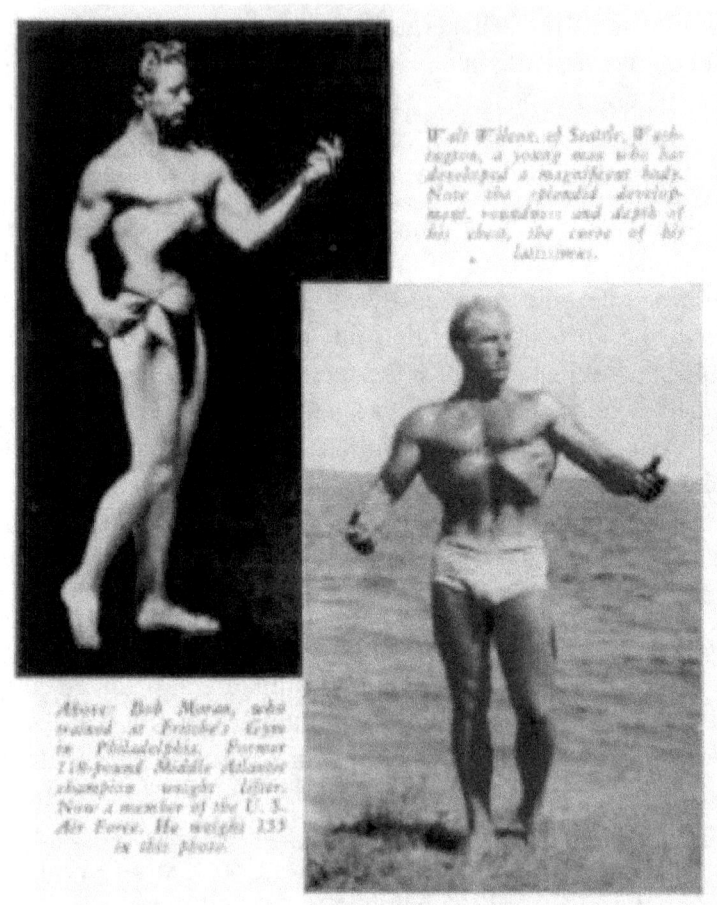

You who read this are interested because you are a body builder—actually a sculptor of your own body. In the beginning, John Grimek possessed sub-average bodily proportions. In his earlier photos it seemed to me that his legs were too short, his torso too long, his waist too broad. He studied his physique, and really chiselled it into the beautiful, statuesque effect that it creates wherever seen at present. He moulded his upper body and limbs, narrowed his waist through proper exercise and proper posture. He deserves more credit than most men for building the superlative physique he now possesses. You want to develop your physique to its fullest. In spite of the musculature you may develop, the size and shapeliness of chest and muscles, it will not present a good appearance because it will be lacking in symmetry and poise unless you make a habit of maintaining the body in the proper position. In every best- built man contest there are men with magnificent muscular developments who are not even placed among the leaders and the prize winners simply because they permit themselves to slump in improper postural positions.

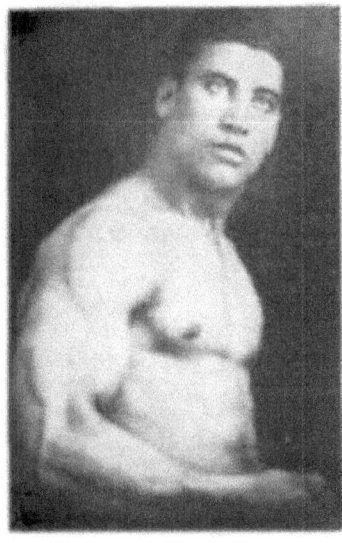
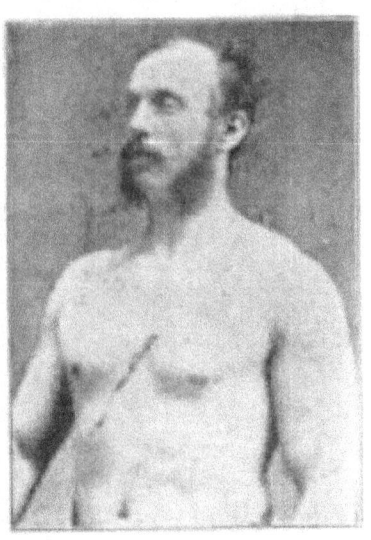

Hassan, of Egypt, former world's champion 181 pound weight lifter.

Richard Pennell, first American to "put up" 200 pound with one hand.

While poor bodily posture is so prevalent, the result of carelessness or ignorance, there are a few who go to the other extreme of walking around constantly with their chests inflated to the limit, with the muscles of their latissimus constantly under tension, with their arms stiffened so that they stand out from the sides at an angle of forty- five degrees. This creates an equally wrong impression; has caused some to believe that weight lifters are so muscle

57

bound that they cannot let their arms hang naturally at the sides. The arms of the most powerfully built men will hang naturally at the sides with the thumbs along the trousers if the latissimus dorsi muscles are not constantly tensed. Hold the chest up and out, the head erect, the shoulders back, but do not keep the chest constantly overinflated.

A study of the anatomical charts in this volume well illustrate why a stooping, faulty posture cramps the heart, lungs and liver and greatly hinders their action. But even more serious ills than result from this cramping of the organs which are high up in the chest occur when a slouching position is habitually maintained. The heart and lungs are upheld by the diaphragm; the liver fits into its under side, but the remainder of the organs in the body do not have so secure a support. The kidneys, stomach, large and small intestines, and important glands, all slip down a little when faulty posture permits the abdomen to be constantly relaxed, and to slip farther and farther forward, as is done when lack of exercise and bad posture continue to be the order of the day.

The stomach will fall as much as two or three inches, resulting in a stretching and constant tension upon the nerves and blood vessels, as well as the tubes which lead to the stomach. The tone of the entire internal system is greatly lowered, and with additional months or years of little use, the muscles become increasingly flabby, fat forms on the outer muscles and about the organs and their action is greatly impaired—much more sluggish than when they are reasonably strong and unimpeded by fatty deposits. For the reasons that I have briefly mentioned, improving posture alone normally results in a quick change for the better in one's innermost feelings.

Habitually bad posture enlarges the waist, diminishes the size of the chest. Our Success Stories, which are received in ever greater abundance, illustrate some startling changes in comparative chest and waist measurements after a short period of training and improvement in posture. Starting training as competitors in the Self-Improvement Contest, March 4th, and training for three months, fifty-two training periods in all, forty-seven-year-old Harry Moss, of Portland, Ore., gained, three inches in normal chest size during this period, and had to change from a 37 to a 40-inch coat. Jerry Charbonneau, St. John, Quebec, reduced his weight 11 pounds during the three months training. Starting with a 37-inch normal chest and a 37-inch normal waist, he had a 45^-inch expanded chest and a 32 Yz-inch waist at the end of the special training period. B. Broodall of Douglass, Arizona, increased his chest from 38 Yz to 42 in eight weeks' time, and he was thirty-five years of age at the time. And these are only several we have selected at random from hundreds of pleased contestants in the Great Strength and Health Self-Improvement Contest.

Many men do not exercise properly. They stand at the pulley weights in a Y. M. C. A. gymnasium, pulling on the weights with their backs curved, their chests flat and their stomachs permitted to sag arid protrude. Good posture and proper breathing are first requisites in proper training, for muscles developed in an improper position are very apt to remain that way at all times. Between exercises most men will walk about for a minute or so. During this period remember your posture. George Hackenschmidt, still renowned as one of the best built big men the world has ever seen, performed between each heavy exercise what he called the Hackenschmidt walk. He would practice full breathing during this period, shoulders back, and draw the waist in with a conscious effort. When he recently made a trip to these shores from his home in France, where he now lives, I had the opportunity to meet him, and at an age past sixty he is still a remarkably well-built man, who at all times maintains good posture.

Proper bar bell exercises, using the widest possible range of muscular movement, from extreme of contraction to extreme of extension, will stretch all the muscles so that it should be easy to form habits of correct posture. The two simple Hackenschmidt exercises were practiced by other famous strength athletes of the day. Hold up the chest and breathe strongly and deeply after the vigorous exertion of the preceding muscle building exercise. This tends to put the spine in the proper position. Pulling in the waist with a constant muscular effort should be a part of every exercise program. Ten times between exercises will be sufficient. If it is not your regular training day, pull in the waist with an effort of the will and the muscles, as many as fifty times in succession in the morning and a similar number at night. Every time you think of it during the day, particularly as you stand or walk about, pull in your waist and hold it there. Even while shaving, remember to practice pulling in your waist. This not only develops the muscles of the abdomen, and compresses the internal works, making the stomach comfortably filled with less food, reducing possibilities of becoming fatter, but massages and invigorates the action of the internal works. Both Eugene Sandow and Louis Cyr spent a great deal of time at pulling in the waist or moving the waist muscles when not engaged in any form of physical exertion.

Before closing this chapter on posture, just another word to help you know when you are maintaining proper posture. Stand with your back to the wall, with your head, hips and shoulders touching the wall. The heels should be one to four inches from the upright surface, depending upon your size and the normal construction of your body. Facing the wall, with your body in the proper position your toes and chest should touch.

A phrase often applied to maintaining correct posture when standing or sitting is to stand or sit " tall." In standing, make yourself as tall as possible without rising upon the toes. Stand with the head up, the chin drawn in slightly, the neck back, and the shoulders back enough that the thumbs touch the seam of the trousers when the arms are hanging naturally at the sides. When long accustomed to poor posture, this will require considerable effort for a time. Plebes or first year men at military academy are required to walk for the first few weeks with their little fingers along the seams of their trousers, the palms front. Try this somewhat exaggerated position. You will see how the shoulders soon can be comfortably maintained in the proper position. As you look at yourself sideways in a full length mirror, standing as you habitually carry yourself, arms hanging naturally, you may find that your thumbs range from six inches to a foot in front of the seams of your trousers.

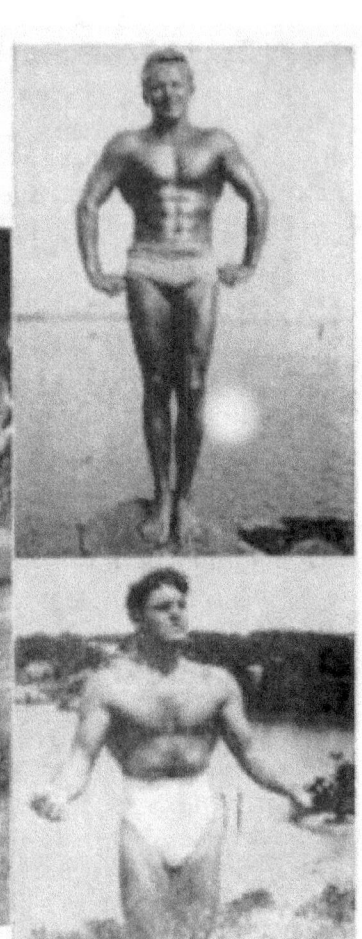

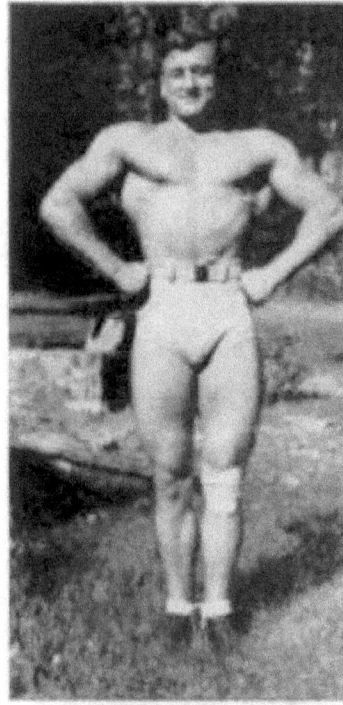

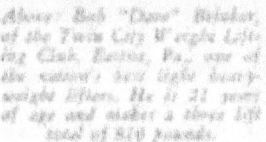

Above: Bob "Dano" Bobolov, of the Twin City Weight Lifting Club, Easton, Pa., one of the nation's best light heavyweight lifters. He is 21 years of age and makes a three lift total of 810 pounds.

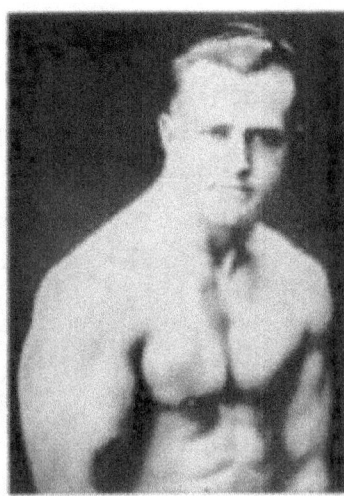

Hold the chest up without straining; this alone should keep the abdomen flat. But for a time it will be wise for you to walk around with it pulled in a bit. This will be easy, for the muscles are becoming stronger and firmer through regular practice of abdominal exercises. Some men wear a tight belt to remind them to stand straight. As the years pass and you order new suits, refuse to have the waist bands made larger. If they are larger it is so easy to eat more or stand less straight, permitting your waistline to grow. Recently I pulled out of the closet and wore for a few days a suit that I wore to the 1932 Olympics. It fits comfortably about the waist in spite of the gains in strength and weight I have made in these eight years. In fact in ordering two suits recently I had to call the tailor's attention to the fact that the waist was a bit loose—to make the new suits an inch smaller. If you find your trouser waist getting tighter, don't permit the tailor to make alterations; make alterations in your living habits and your posture.

Maintain the spine in as straight a position as possible, particularly the lower part or small of the back. Some men permit themselves to become " sway backed " by going on year after year standing in a faulty position. The legs have some bearing on proper posture—stand and complete each stride with the knees straight; keep the toes nearly straight to the front. Europeans have a tendency to toe out, American Indians to toe in; straight to the front is the best way.

While your exercise periods will average three or four hours a week a half hour a day, you'll have sixteen hours a day or more during which you are up and about. Proper posture during these hours will not only aid you to keep the gains in chest size that you have made, but help you increase these gains. Spending these long hours slumping about in sitting or standing will not rob you of all that you have gained, but it will retard your much-desired gains in chest size. Therefore remember to sit tall, for more of the majority of people's time is spent sitting than standing or walking. Keep the spine straight in sitting. When it is necessary to lean forward, lean from the hips, keeping your back as straight as possible. Keep the feet flat upon the floor. In sleeping, spend as much time stretched out as possible rather than with the body in distorted positions.

It's wise to take an inventory of your physical condition, including your posture, at times. Good posture, as we will constantly reiterate, means better health and far better and a much more admired appearance of the well-built man. There is a favorable contrast between chest and waist which causes the former to appear even larger than it is. When taking this physical inventory of yourself be sure that your shoulders are not rounded, your chest flattened or your abdomen protruding.

"Getting Into Condition"

WHEN the average man runs as little as one block to catch a train, he becomes completely winded. Perhaps you have learned this about your own physical condition. You were a bit late, well within sight of the station, but at least a quarter mile to go and less than two minutes until train time. You had been catching this train every morning for the last year or so, had had to hurry at times, but never more than a fast walk before. But this time you had the alternative of picking up and setting your feet down a little faster by actually running to make the train or waiting until the next one which would make you late to business.

If you were doing a fair amount of physical work, your legs were in pretty good condition, but you felt real distress after completing your run to the train. After you entered the car you were panting for breath and felt well-nigh exhausted. Your distress continued long after the extreme exertion was ended. You continued to be completely winded, out of breath, yet your legs which seemed to be the chief motivating force were not tired. This phenomenon probably puzzled you. Your legs which apparently did the work were not tired yet your lungs were panting, your heart pumping, which would lead you to believe that they were not strong.

Your heart and lungs had become accustomed to performing certain work. When called upon to do much more they protested strongly, and many long minutes were required before a condition of normal heart and lung action was regained. The unusual action of the legs required much greater quantities of oxygen; the heart and lungs were laboring to supply them. An oxygen debt had piled up during your enforced run, and even after the muscles were no longer in use, as you rested upon the cushions, the heart and lungs were hard at work to pay that debt, and only when the debt was paid could they return to normal operation and you were once again comfortable.

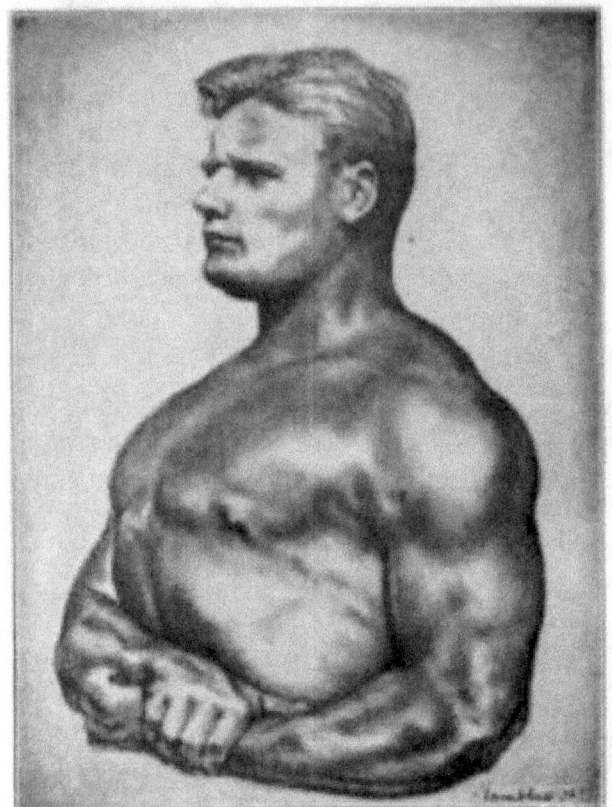

Drawing by Gord Venables of Walter Podalak. Walter, long famed for his development and strength, former holder of the world's dead weight lift record at 643 pounds, is now a professional wrestler.

You have noticed athletes " warming up " before a run or a contest. Paavo Nurmi, the great Finnish runner, or Glenn Cunningham, the Kansas youth who bettered some of his records, would sometimes run one or two miles to warm up before the actual start of the race. This warming up loosened the muscles, but most of all it speeded i he action of the heart and lungs, so that they adjusted themselves to the increased demands which were to be made upon them during the race. In running for the train, if you had been able to start slowly and were at least a little accustomed to running, you would have obtained your second wind and not arrived at the train so near complete exhaustion.

When a man starts out in the beginning of the season to practice cross-country, track, football, or even crew he commences to run a little. He runs a little more each day, and with the passing days his internal works become accustomed to the increased exertions demanded of them, so that they deliver increased quantities of the blood sugar and oxygen required to keep the muscles in operation. Constant practice, improving the action of the important internal works, makes the difference between the great fatigue and breathlessness you or any other untrained man experience from suddenly running to catch a train and the five to ten miles that trained runners traverse so easily. They have built endurance in heart and lungs as well as limbs.

The average man if he swims the length of a normal pool —75 feet—unless he is a good swimmer and has practiced at least a fair amount of swimming in recent months, will arrive at the end of the pool breathless. Yet a trained swimmer can continue for hours without breathlessness. He has learned to breathe fully while in the water. It is easier to draw in sufficient breath at each double stroke than it is to exhale fully enough to provide enough fresh air for subsequent strokes.

Jumping rope is difficult for the average man; he soon becomes breathless. Yet men have skipped rope without a miss for hour after hour, simply because they become accustomed to the exertion. Deep knee bending with one's bodyweight is difficult for the average man. I have seen corpulent men and women who did not possess enough strength to arise once from the low position of the deep knee bend, and have seen many others who became so breathless from a few bends that they could not continue. Yet men who have specialized in repetition deep knee bends have continued for thousands of bends. The difference is becoming accustomed to the movements and simultaneously strengthening the body inside and out so that the desired movement can be continued for a lengthy period.

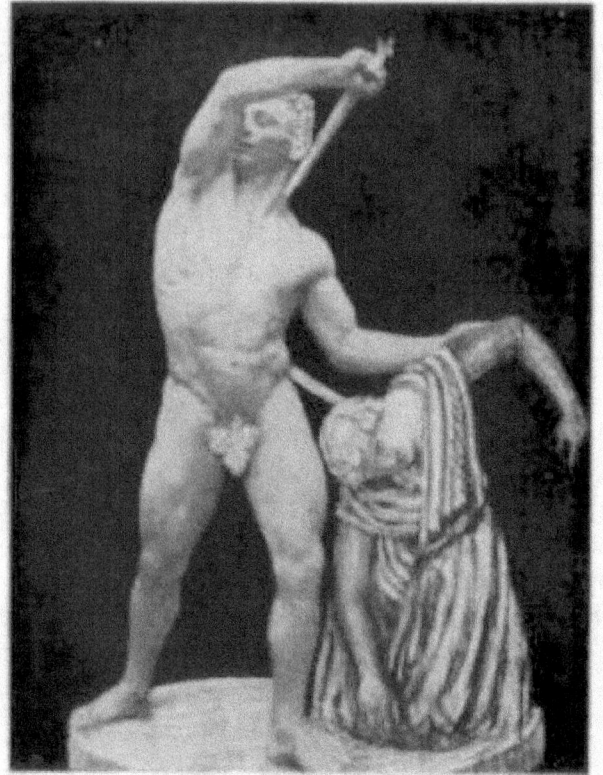

Otto Arco, one of the world's most famous strength and development figures, posed for this famous work of statuary.

While deep breathing alone will not give you the ability to swim far, run far, or skip rope thousands of times, unless you practice these particular exercises, the deep breathing (particularly when coupled with vigorous exercise which places demands upon the body) will be highly beneficial. Deep breathing when no exertion is made will not improve your endurance but deep breathing coupled with vigorous exercise will make you not only stronger and healthier but a great deal more enduring. Deep breathing practiced during your progressive training periods will greatly increase the capacity of your chest and its strength, but if you wish to excel at physical pastimes such as I have enumerated you must practice these particular sports or exercises.

The total quantity of work demanded of the muscles produces general breathlessness. Muscular fatigue is local, as can easily be proven if you determine how many times you can press a twenty-five-pound weight overhead with one hand, but if you see how many times you can deep knee bend with one hundred pounds then you create the general effect of breathlessness because you have brought all the muscles into action. When work is too light to produce breathlessness, only fatigue, you cannot expect to obtain favorable results in building chest size, strength or endurance.

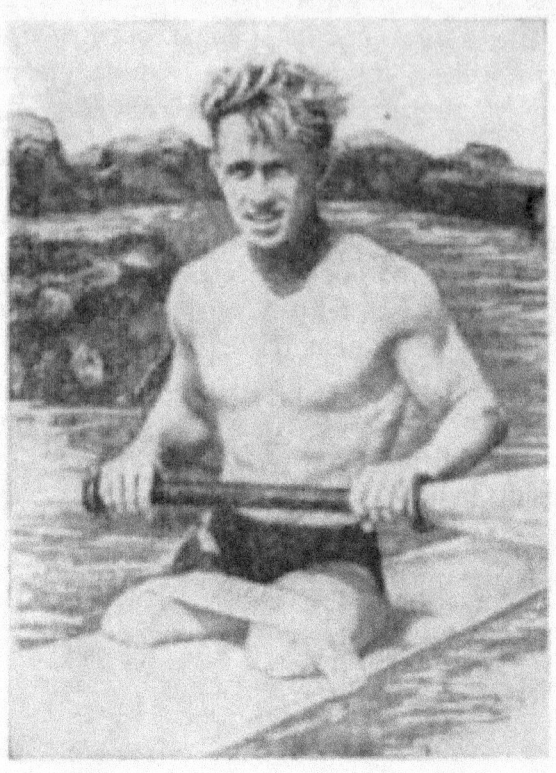

In direct contrast, if you exert to the limit of their ability the larger muscles of the body, the muscles can become tired before a condition of breathlessness is created. As, for instance, in very heavy dead weight lifting or deep knee bending, perhaps seven movements can be made, which are all one could expect from the muscles if a weight is very heavy, before a condition of breathlessness will result. Therefore it is necessary in endeavoring to build the chest with heavy exercise to continue the movements to a point where great breathlessness results. While some physical trainers recommend thirty or even more deep knee bends I do not favor so many, preferring not to exceed fifteen bends as a muscle- building exercise—twenty as a breathing exercise. If more bends are practiced, and the movement is continuous, the weight must feel light to begin and then toward the end it becomes difficult enough. This sort of movement builds endurance rather than strength in muscles and greatest lung capacity. On the other hand it is not possible to use a great weight for enough movements to really cause enforced breathing. That's why I recommend the heavy and light system for those who desire to build great strength in muscles, tendons and ligaments—at least ten movements for muscle building, and up to twenty to enlarge the chest.

Most men who have established high records in deep knee bending with heavy weights perform a series of strength feats rather than continuous deep knee bending. They take three or even more breaths between each bend. Weldon Bullock, the first seventeen-year-old boy in the history of weight lifting to clean and jerk three hundred pounds, followed this system. In 1933, at the national weight lifting championships in Chicago, he made the highest clean and jerk of all those present with his lift of 309. He was seventeen years of age at the time. In deep knee bending he would perform as many as thirty, and breathed in such an exaggerated manner between bends that neighbors from a half block around would congregate at the doors of the training quarters, probably to see who was being tortured to death. Between each bend he would breathe deeply and expel the air from his lungs with a " huh, hoh, huh " which could be heard for a block. It is true that heavy exertion Continued for long periods such as Bullock did it, with three or four deep breaths between each movement, will enlarge the chest, but we have so many other desired ends to obtain from physical training that I do not generally recommend such a program. It is not a part of the regular York courses, but is recommended by myself or other York instructors to the specialist who is striving primarily for increased chest size.

During heavy deep knee bending it is not too difficult to inhale sufficient air, but as in swimming it is hard to expel the air which has passed through the lungs. That was the reason for the great effort Bullock expended in expelling the used air from his lungs.

I will repeat a number of times through the chapters in this book the important rule that increased chest size only results from exercises which cause breathlessness by making great demands upon the muscles. While it is possible to create a condition of breathlessness by holding one's breath, or even remaining under water for a long period, this is not a recommended way to build the chest, for as previously mentioned it also creates a strain upon heart and lungs.

Any man in reasonably good condition can run evenly and at a moderate pace for a quarter or half mile or even farther without becoming especially breathless. He will be breathing more forcefully, for the heart and chest, having so much more work to do, naturally will be operating more powerfully, but if he runs faster, or uphill, then real effort is demanded of the internal works. Jumping into the air or stair climbing greatly adds to the effort expended. I have always enjoyed reading about athletes and athletics. I have seen in action, for a great many years, nearly every well-known athlete in every branch of sport. I am a lover of all sports, have taken part in most of them, really enjoy seeing the champions in any sport in action. Weight lifting or weight training is my first love, for I realize that it is the finest form of training and produces more physical benefits in less time than any other line of physical endeavor. But I do see other sports when I can.

I believe I have seen every great sprinter for the last score of years in action at the championships or the Olympic games. I casually knew one of these sprinters and had read of his exploits. lie was the national champion one year when a group of America's best track and field athletes went upon a world tour at the request of various governments. This young man excelled the best sprinters in every country in which he competed. He was in his prime, in the very pink of condition, when he came to Egypt. One day they went on a visit to the great pyramids and there this sprinter learned of the record which was held by one of the Egyptian guides for running to the top of the pyramid. The American sprinter thought that he could improve upon that record and offered to bet his companions. The pyramid was high, the steps almost too great for a man to actually run up them. The American reached the top in faster time than any other man in the history of the world attained, but he paid dearly for it. He drove his heart and lungs, unaccustomed to such work, and his muscles past the point of normal fatigue. He could hardly walk from the scene of his exploit unassisted, so cramped were his muscles and so labored was the action of his sorely tried heart and lungs. Some time after that he experienced a physical collapse, so that when I have seen him at various national A. A. U. meetings he still walks with the aid of crutches. More than likely the straining effort he put forth in Egypt resulted ultimately in his physical collapse. Had he been able to gradually accustom himself to the unusual exertion of running up the pyramids he would not have suffered so, physically.

Gradually building the ability to breathe deeply and forcefully, making physical demands upon the body which create breathlessness, and abetting these demands through proper, enforced breathing will build bigger, deeper chests, and invariably the man with the biggest chest will be more enduring than the man with a flatter chest—not in movements of light endurance, for men with small chests could build sufficient endurance to run a score or more of miles. Indians' weighing less than a hundred pounds have run a hundred miles; frail men and women have ridden a bicycle for hundreds of miles or walked a hundred miles. But they would not have power and endurance combined, which is much to be desired and striven for.

If you consider your own friends you must know some vital, enduring men who have big, deep chests, and you must know some men with smaller, shallow chests. The man with the bigger chest invariably will possess more endurance than the thinner person. The thin person will work on nervous energy and having less weight to carry may continue all day, but cannot keep this up day after day to the extent that the vital big-chested man can. The big-chested man continues his efforts on muscular power alone, husbanding his physical resources, so that he is more placid in disposition, more tranquil in mind, while the thinner, small- chested man works on nerve force and finally pays.

The Treasure Chest of Life

TREASURE chest—what thoughts of pieces of eight, gold ornaments, pearls, diamonds and other jewels that must conjure—particularly in the youthful mind. Who hasn't dreamed at some time in his life of searching for buried treasure, perhaps the treasures reputed to have been buried by the bold pirates of old upon the islands of the Caribbean! Who hasn't dreamed a little of Arabian nights tales, or given some thought to the storied caves and warehouses, filled with treasure chests, of Indian potentates believed to be the wealthiest men in this wide world.

This form of treasure has much material value, intrinsic worth past belief, but what original owner of this fabulous wealth when he finds himself ill and aging would Jiot give it all for a few more years of life? Strong, vigorous years, when a man should be at the zenith of all his faculties. No man has a need for more than a moderate amount of this world's goods; one can only eat so much, sleep in one bed and, to remain strong and healthy, can only participate in a few moderate pleasures. It's a case of when one can eat a horse he can't afford it and when he can afford it he can't eat it.

So getting down to real values we find that the greatest value of all is how we feel, and this is controlled by the condition and action of our internal organs. I have titled this chapter in what some may believe to be an odd manner to bring out the point that the real human treasure chest is your own chest. That's the only treasure chest that really matters to you. How you feel, the length and happiness of your life, is controlled by the organs in that chest more than any others. Yes, the human chest box constitutes the human treasure chest of health, strength and vitality.

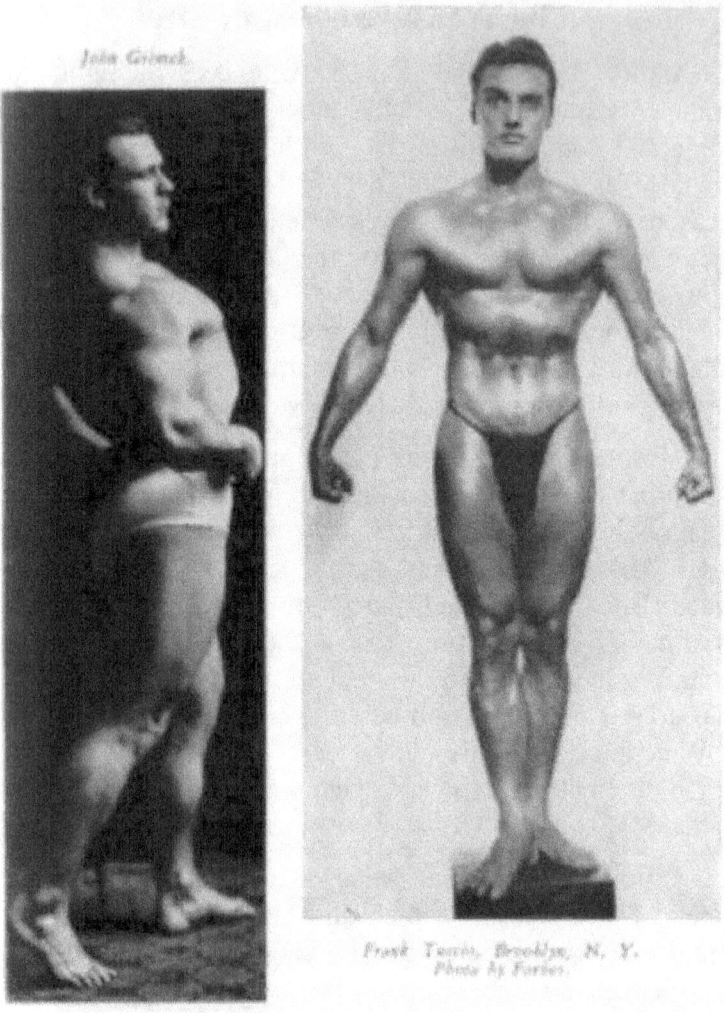

John Grimek

Frank Torin, Brooklyn, N. Y.
Photo by Forbes

So many articles have been written concerning the importance of other muscles and other muscle groups, of other organs, of the various parts of the body and its numerous appendages, organs, glands, cells, so many articles stressing the importance of arms, back, legs, sides, lower back, abdomen, that it would be natural for the reader to become perplexed as to just what portion of the body is really most important. All are important, for each part must depend on some other portion of the body. All are parts of a whole, each depending upon the other like the links of a chain, and when one part fails, just as in the breaking of a chain, future life is impaired or ended depending upon the importance and function of the organ which has failed.

As you continue with this book, I believe you will agree with its author, that the contents of the human treasure chest of life, the chest or rib box, to which so little thought is ordinarily given, are the organs which are most necessary to the well being, strength, and endurance of the. body. The important parts it contains have the most beneficial relationship to your physical well being. As we delve farther into the study of the organs contained in the thoracic region of the chest you will become thoroughly convinced of the importance of chest development in the production of health, strength and longevity.

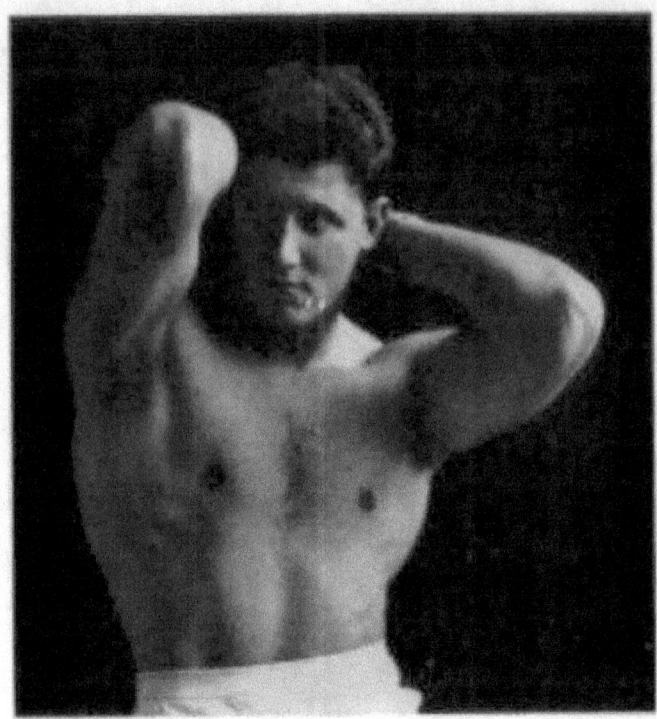

Jack "Human Guinea Pig" Cooper, of the York Bar Bell Club. Jack is now 19 years of age and in his most recent lifting made 243 press, 275 snatch, 353 clean and jerk, total 873. In one year and a half he built his 5 ft. 4½-inch body from 135 pounds to 212, and the great strength indicated by his weight lifting total.

There is no other part of the body which contains organs so necessary to the business of living as does the chest. The chief organs encased in this bony framework are the heart and lungs. Among the necessary functions these rank at the head of the list. While we could live indefinitely after the injury or removal of some of the organs, life would last only moments when the action of the lungs ceases and only seconds when the heart fails. I intend to write considerable concerning the importance of the anatomy of the chest, and the organs it contains. I hope you will be patient with this discussion and realize its importance. Make a careful study of the anatomy of this most important part of your body so that you will desire to develop the chest and all it contains until you have a real treasure chest of life. No repetition I could make would be too frequent concerning this subject, for nothing can be more important than for every man to realize the necessity of having knowledge of the body, particularly the part of the body we are now discussing, and putting forth untiring, ceaseless efforts to develop these parts to their limit.

A well-developed chest is not only attractive to look at, not only extremely useful in work or athletics, but its internal strength and efficiency of operation will prevent and overcome most any chest and lung troubles. Courage and confidence are possessed by men and women who have well-developed chests, for they are able to surmount any physical difficulties which may beset them as well as to avoid or overcome lung troubles such as consumption, commonly called tuberculosis, asthma, catarrh, bronchitis, weak lungs, pleurisy, pulmonary diseases, pneumonia and similar forms of premature death.

Our Success Letters published monthly in Strength and Health magazine cite many cases of men who have overcome serious disorders such as those enumerated in, the previous paragraph. Perhaps the most outstanding case is that of Roger Eells of Ohio. Some years ago Roger, as the result of an accident when an airplane propeller struck and crushed his chest, found himself in an advanced stage of consumption. One lung was completely collapsed; the other nearly so. He was given just three months to live. Naturally under these circumstances his insurance company was forced to pay him total disability charges. When he first received these dire reports he sold his interest in his business, and started out to see something of life during the short months he had before him. But he was made of stern stuff physically as well as in determination as he later proved.

At the end of three months he had not passed along as was' so freely prophesied and began to wonder if there mightn't be something he could do to overcome his difficulty. He began reading all the physical training and medical books he could obtain—books such as this—and decided that physical exercise might be the proper solution. He wrote to me and in the beginning told me that he would take my course if I would guarantee that he would gain twenty pounds. His weight had dropped to 121 pounds from 150, which he had weighed prior to the serious accident in which he was involved. This left him little more than skin and bones.

I refused to make the guarantee of twenty pounds' gain, but cited numerous cases of those who had gained weight even under the most adverse circumstances, and enumerated a few others who had not gained weight but had attained perfect health and two or three times average strength. He was convinced enough to make his start with the four York bar bell and dumbell courses. In a remarkably short time he had gained weight: to 132 pounds, to 145, and after a few short months to 162. At this weight he presented a well-built, handsome appearance, though he had sufficient height to require more weight if he were to be considered really well built.

It was freely prophesied at this time that, while he had improved in bodyweight and appearance, the strain he had placed upon his weakened organs would no doubt cause him to drop dead most any day. But the days passed and finally Roger was completely cured. A story appeared in Strength and Health magazine concerning his rise from the shadow of death to a position of usefulness, health, strength and happiness in this world.

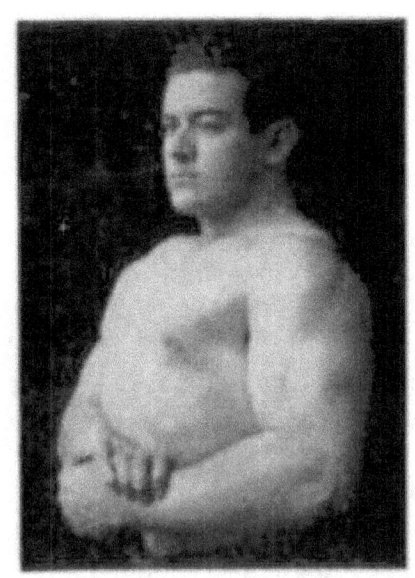

A fine photo of fads Hoskins, which shows his 50-inch chest and 18-inch arms to splendid advantage.

The story was widely read and created quite a furore in various circles. I was cited by the Federal Trade Commission for unfair advertising. One of my competitors claimed that Roger had benefited from his system of training, because he had read his books. The Federal Trade Commission thought that I had exaggerated his condition. The Federal Trade attorneys had hearings in Washington, Philadelphia, and York, Pa. Roger Eells expressed a willingness to come here and prove that a transformation had truly been made through York bar bell training. The Federal Trade lawyer said, "Mr. Eells, didn't you write to Mr. Blank about your condition?" Roger agreed that he did. The lawyer said, "That's all I want to know. Just testify to that when you get on the witness stand." And on the stand Mr. Eells amplified his statement a bit by saying, "Yes, I wrote to Mr. Blank, but he tried to discourage me. He told me that exercise in my condition was not only useless but actually dangerous and would prob.ably end my life prematurely. But Mr. Hoffman encouraged me and I followed his system with the results you see upon my own person and have read about."

And then he produced doctors' reports prepared at the depth of his physical debility to provt that his condition was as we had advertised and that later he was completely- cured. Roger Eells followed the four York courses exactly as they were offered for a time; then he included with his training a great deal of lung and chest-developing exercises. He specialized in the deep knee bend—breathing squats as this system is so often phrased—taking three or four deep breaths between each bend, squatting on full lungs, and continuing with this movement to a fairly high number of repetitions. The stiff-legged dead weight lift and the two arm pull over were his other specialties. He not only over-came his condition, but built a splendid healthy body and now he is teaching bar bell training and is a source of great good for others throughout the world.

As an aftermath to all of his hard labor, his insurance company heard that he was cured, had him tested before their own physicians and discontinued any form of benefit payments. Later Roger was scheduled to tour the country as a lecturer for the Tuberculosis League, but he was pre-vented from doing this as some felt that he was the excep-tion rather than the rule. He had benefited greatly, they agreed, had been completely cured, but, so they reasoned, some other man might injure himself through such ex-ercises.

But the fact does remain that exercises such as are offered in the chapters of this volume will overcome the majority of lung ills and will build such strength, health and resist-ance to pulmonary diseases that most men and women who practice the movements will go through life without the slightest inconvenience from the common cold. It is many years since I have had a cold and I attribute my freedom from this common ill to the practice of chest exercises such as I am offering. It has been said that there is no way to entirely cure the ordinary cold. If this were true it would be necessary for you to resign yourself to spending the rest of your life being annoyed with constant coughing, sniffling and hacking. But the human body was designed to operate perfectly. It has within itself the ability to cure or overcome all injuries or ills. And the lungs, when given the proper opportunity, given sufficient " living space" and fortified and strengthened through general body-conditioning exercises, particularly deep breathing exercises in conjunction with progressive exercise, will build such resistance to pulmonary difficulties that you will not be annoyed by these common, but nevertheless annoying, troubles in the future.

To cite the case of another prominent physical culturist, Ray Van Cleef, who recently wrote as follows: "Like many youngsters, during the period of adolescence my growth was too rapid in proportion to my vitality. By the time I reached the age of twelve I was in a run-down condition, and was considerably underweight. Being in such a frail state of health I proved an easy victim to sickness. In the course of having frequent illnesses that year, I contracted a chest cold. Had I been in good health I would have been able to overcome it without any serious complications. But, in spite of receiving proper care under medical supervision, my system was too weak to combat the ravages of the disease. The result was an attack of pneumonia. After a long siege of this critical sickness I recuperated. With my vitality being further weakened by this illness, however, I contracted pneumonia again before the year was over. This second attack proved even more serious than the first in that the after-effects left me with a fluid deposit in my lungs which had to be removed. My doctor was gravely concerned over my health and feared that I might become a victim of tuberculosis unless some measures were employed to build up my vitality and increase my resistance.

He prescribed a series of deep breathing exercises for me to practice. It was there and then that my active association with physical culture commenced.

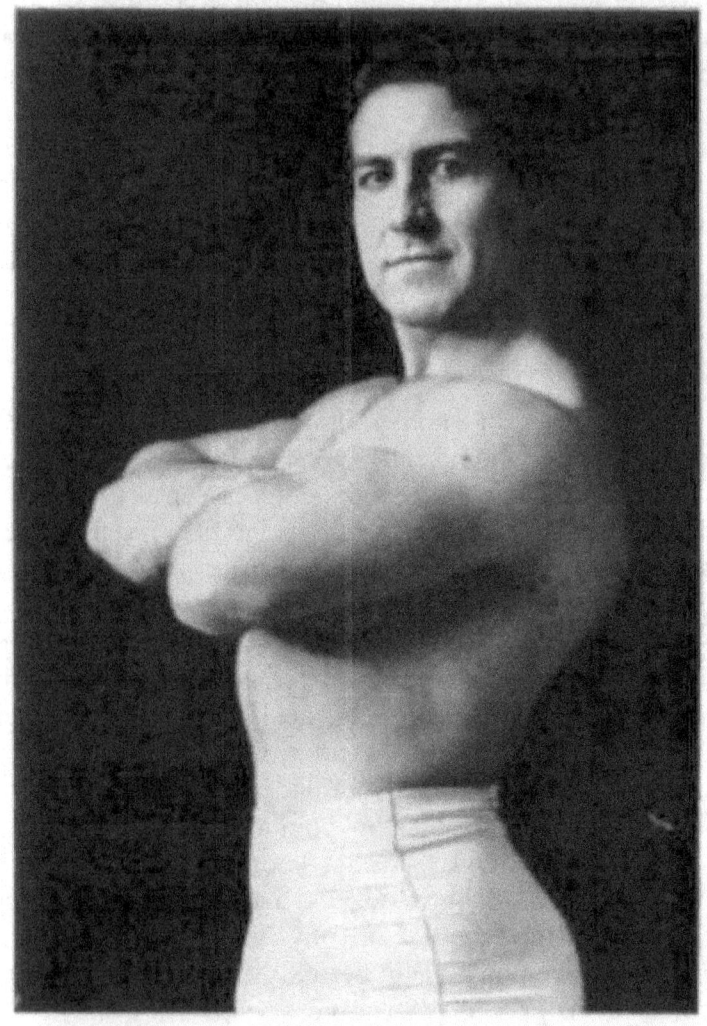

Tony Terlazzo, of the York Bar Bell Club, long famous as the world's best weight lifter, a 132-pound lifter for some years, national champion in this class in 1932 and 1936. He won the 1936 Olympic title and then surpassed by winning the world's 148-pound championship the following year. He has won more honors than any other one weight lifter. United States champion 8 times, champion of North America every year, Olympic champion, and world's champion of 1936-37-38-39 and 40.

" The beneficial results that I obtained from even these elementary exercises were so encouraging that once I fully recuperated I was anxious to further advance in my physical culture endeavors; so I employed more advanced methods of training. The rebuilding of my health firmly convinced me that the only way to enjoy a vigorous state of health and to avoid sickness was by adhering to the physical culture mode of life.

" Now that I have briefly discussed my state of poor health and susceptibility to colds prior to the commencement of practicing physical culture, I wish to relate a few facts in regard to my experience with colds after I had acquired vigorous health. During my school days I did considerable running as a member of a cross-country team. In practicing this sport in the late fall season there were many days when we ran the course under such adverse weather conditions as mist, rain and even snow on a number of occasions. Many times the temperature was below freezing, yet all we wore were a scanty pair of trunks and a sleeveless shirt. Needless to say, my parents were worried that I would ' catch my death of cold.' But quite to the contrary I did not acquire even a sniffle, let alone a cold, and neither did the other members of the team. In fact, being in good physical condition at this time, the frigid, damp air served as an invigorating tonic."

Mr. Van Cleef goes on to explain that with more advanced physical training methods, during which he became particularly famed for his strength and hand-balancing ability, he has not had the slightest cold for years. His case is similar to that of hundreds of other weight lifters and strength athletes whom I number among my personal acquaintances. We have plenty of proof to offer that nature did not intend that the human body should be constantly ailing, suffering from a never-ending stream of minor or major ills, but that it should continue without disease, which of course means perfect health.

While deep breathing exercises, developing the chest and lungs to the fullest extent, provide the best means to avoid or overcome pulmonary diseases which range from the common cold to tuberculosis, other health laws should be included in the mode of living: a regular course of all-around body-conditioning exercises, eating proper food, well-balanced meals at mealtimes only, sufficient rest or relaxation, and the proper frame of mind. While these are our four major health rules so often written about—they are the best rules to follow to avoid chest ills of all sorts—to these may be added a few more important rules such as avoiding contact with those who are suffering from colds. When really strong and vigorous you need not fear infection from another, but don't expose yourself needlessly unless you must. During the Great War, I spent the winter of 1918- 1919 in a mud hole which was known as " St. Agony " to the soldiers who were there, and I believe that at least a million soldiers of the A. E. F. were in that camp at one time or another. It was at St. Agnain, France, and was a casual camp. Men returning to their organizations from the hospital went through that camp for equipment. Prisoners being returned from Germany passed through that camp and remained there for a time. It rained constantly; we waded through endless mud, lived in cold, damp tents, and two squads of grave diggers were busy for long hours every day. Firing of guns over the graves of departed comrades and the blowing of taps were heard several times each day. But I didn't even have a sniffle as Ray Van Cleef mentioned in his own case. Certainly it was resistance to disease of any sort which had been engendered by physical training, particularly deep breathing in my regular exercise before and during the war, and in athletic competition, that maintained me through that winter in perfect health while so many unfortunates were buried there.

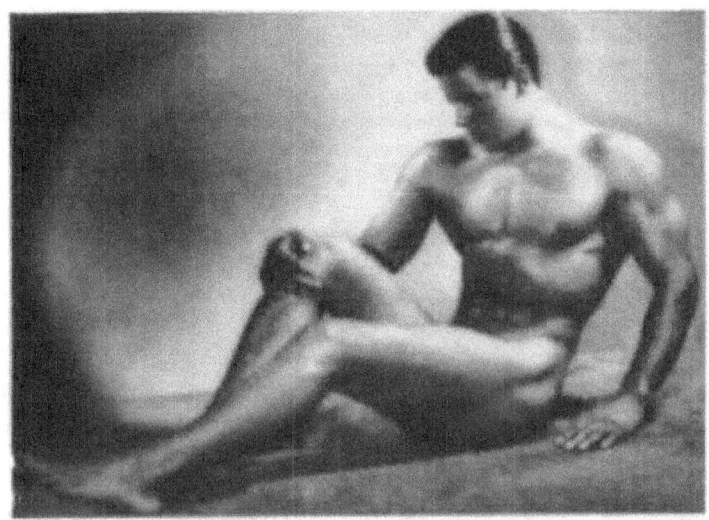
Arnold Dublin, of Santa Monica, Cal., another famous York Bar Bell man.

Another rule to follow is to avoid constipation. Breathe through the nose. In each nostril are hairs designed to strain the air and warm it before it passes to the lungs. If you breathe through the mouth, the cold, often smoky or dirty air is drawn directly into the lungs. When possible, work in well-ventilated rooms, which are properly heated and of course insist on these conditions at home, where you can more easily control them. Drink sufficient water; have well- ventilated bedrooms at night. This does not necessarily mean wide open windows with the snow blowing in upon us as we thought was best in our childhood. Two windows in a room, not weather stripped, leak as much air as could come in freely through an opening a foot square. Do not have the air in your home too dry. Water in pans upon registers or radiators will provide the additional humidity the moist passages of the nasal passages and the lungs require. Keep yourself clean with daily baths and frequent washing of hands and face and drink an ample supply of water each day. These may seem like minor rules in some cases, but they are all important.

And above all include with your regular training plenty of breathing exercises with weights.

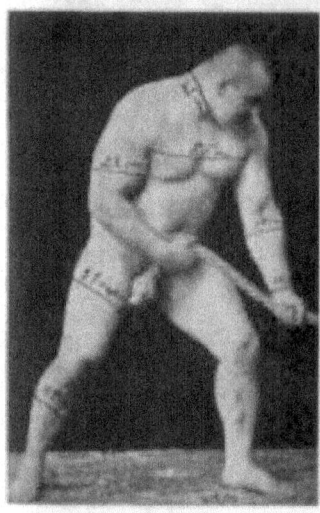
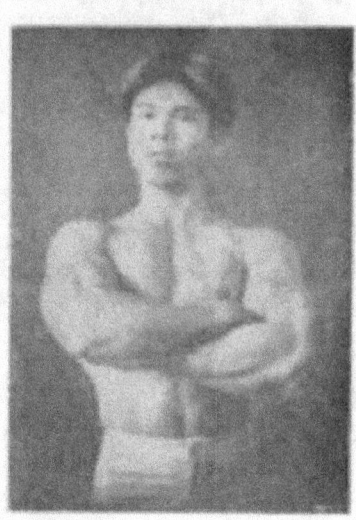

There are so many reasons for building your rib box, your lungs and the muscles on the outside of the chest, that any time spent in developing the chest inside and out will be time well spent. There will be a direct connection between these exercises, a direct proportion of improved health, increased strength, greater vitality and endurance —a glorious muscular development and a complete freedom from all ills and distressing conditions of the chest region.

I am sorry that I cannot give you a big healthy chest. You'll have to win. that for yourself. All I can do is tell you the superior way, outline the best exercises and a mode of living which provide the quickest and easiest way to derive the desired ends of a powerful, healthy chest. You will first of all have to desire to have this big healthy chest, and then have sufficient persistence to continue with your endeavors until you have a chest which compares favorably with the men whose photos appear in this book, and numerous other outstanding physical specimens whose pictures could not be shown as the pages of a book are not unlimited.

I am trying to include the most important pieces of advice somewhere in this book, trying to avoid repetition, and perhaps this is as good a place as any to tell you that first you must aspire to have this big chest, then be willing to perspire to obtain it. You will require constant inspiration, so keep this book around where you can go through its pages at frequent intervals, absorbing the knowledge it contains and being encouraged by the photos of men with splendid physiques who have succeeded in obtaining their outstanding development through the practice of the advice I am offering you.

It is a good plan to cut out photos of big-chested men; place these upon large cards—frame them if you wish— and have them on the walls of your training quarters. By keeping your goal of a perfect body—particularly a big healthy chest—constantly in mind, it will first of all give you something definite to strive for, but most of all provide a source of encouragement for you.

Before launching on a special chest-developing program you should measure yourself, and obtain a before picture if possible. You will be thrilled by the improvement you make and it will be a source of encouragement to some other man who is seeking increased strength, health and development. You will be surprised at the tale the tape measure will tell you in a few weeks of regular training, and at the change in your appearance as shown fleetingly by the mirror and permanently by photos.

Make haste slowly. Don't try to go too fast. Start gradually; wait until the muscles and the lungs, too, are accustomed to the increased work required of them before going ahead with increased vigor. I wish you all sorts of success in acquiring an admiration-creating chest development of which you can be proud.

Anatomical Description of the Lungs

IN the two lateral chambers of the thoracic cavity are the two cone-shaped organs we know as the lungs. They are separated from each other by the heart and other contents of the mediastinum. The outer surface of each lung is convex, a concave base to fit over the convex portion of the diaphragm, and extending about an inch and a half above the level of the sternal end of the first rib is an apex. The pulmonary artery connects each lung with the heart and trachea, the pulmonary vein, bronchial arteries and veins, and a number of other parts constitute the root of the lungs. The hilum or vertical notch is located on the inner surface. This provides a passage to the structures which form the root of the lung. Below and in front of the hilum there is a deep concavity, called the cardiac impression, which accommodates the heart. It is larger and deeper on the left than on the right lung, because the heart extends farther to the left side.

The right lung is the larger and heavier of the two. It has greater breadth than the left, owing to the inclination of the heart to the left side, and it is shorter by one inch, because the diaphragm rises higher on the right side to ac-commodate the liver. The right lung is divided by fissures into three lobes, which are titled superior, middle and in-ferior. The left lung is smaller, narrower and longer than the right and is divided into just two lobes, the inferior and the superior.

The material of which the lungs are formed is porous, soft and spongy. It floats in water owing to the presence of air which crepitates when handled. The lungs consist of bronchial tubes and their terminal dilations, numerous blood vessels, lymphatics, nerves and a great many fine, elastic, connective tissues which bind all parts together. Each lobe of the lung is composed of many lobules, and into each lobule a bronchiole enters and * terminates in an atrium. Each atrium presents a series of air cells. In this way the amount of surface exposed to the air and covered by the capillaries is so immensely increased that it is estimated the entire inner surface of the lungs amounts to about ninety square meters, more than one hundred times the skin surface of the entire body.

There are two sets of blood vessels in the lungs. First the branches of the pulmonary artery, which transports the blood to the lungs to be aerated and the branches of the bronchial arteries which bring blood for nutritive purposes. Immediately beneath the layer of flat cells, and lodged in the elastic connective tissue, is a very close plexus of capillaries, and the air reaching the alveoli by the bronchial tubes is separated from the blood by the capillaries, which coalesce to form larger branches. These run through the substance of the lung, communicate with other branches, and form larger vessels, which accompany the arteries and bronchial tubes to the hilum. Finally the pulmonary veins open into the left auricle.

The branches of the bronchial arteries supply blood to the long substance—the bronchial tubes, coats of the blood vessels, the lymph nodes and the pleura. The bronchial veins formed at the root of each lung receive veins which correspond to the branches of the bronchial arteries.

Each lung is enclosed in a serous sac—the pleura, one layer of which is closely adherent to the walls of the chest and diaphragm; the other closely covers the lung. The two layers of the pleural sacs, moistened by serum, are normally in close contact, and the so-called pleural cavity is a potential rather than an actual cavity. They move easily upon one another and prevent the friction that would otherwise occur between the lungs and the walls of the chest with every respiration. If the surface of the pleura becomes roughened as occurs in inflammation (pleurisy) more or less friction results and the sound produced by this friction can be heard if the ear is applied to the breast. In health, only a small amount of fluid is secreted and its absorption by the lymphatics almost keeps pace with its secretion, so that normally the amount of serum is very small. In pleurisy the amount may be considerably increased, due to the extra activity of the irritated secretory cells and excessive transudation from the congested blood vessels. The amount may be sufficient to separate the two layers of the pleura, thus changing the potential pleural cavity into an actual one. This is known as pleurisy with effusion. The mediastinum, or interpleural space, lies between the right and left pleura in the median plane of the chest. It extends from the sternum to the spinal column and is entirely filled with thoracic viscera, namely the heart, aorta and its branches, pulmonary artery and veins, with other parts, various veins, lymph nodes and nerves.

The main purpose of respiration is to supply the cells of the body with oxygen and rid them of the excess carbon dioxide which results from the oxidation. It also helps to equalize the temperature of the body and get rid of excess water. To accomplish these purposes three processes are necessary:

1. Breathing. The process of breathing may be subdivided into inspiration or breathing in, and expiration or breathing out. 2. External respiration. This includes two processes— external oxygen supply or the passage of oxygen from the alveoli of the lungs to the blood and external carbon dioxide elimination or the passage of carbon dioxide from the blood into the alveoli of the lungs.

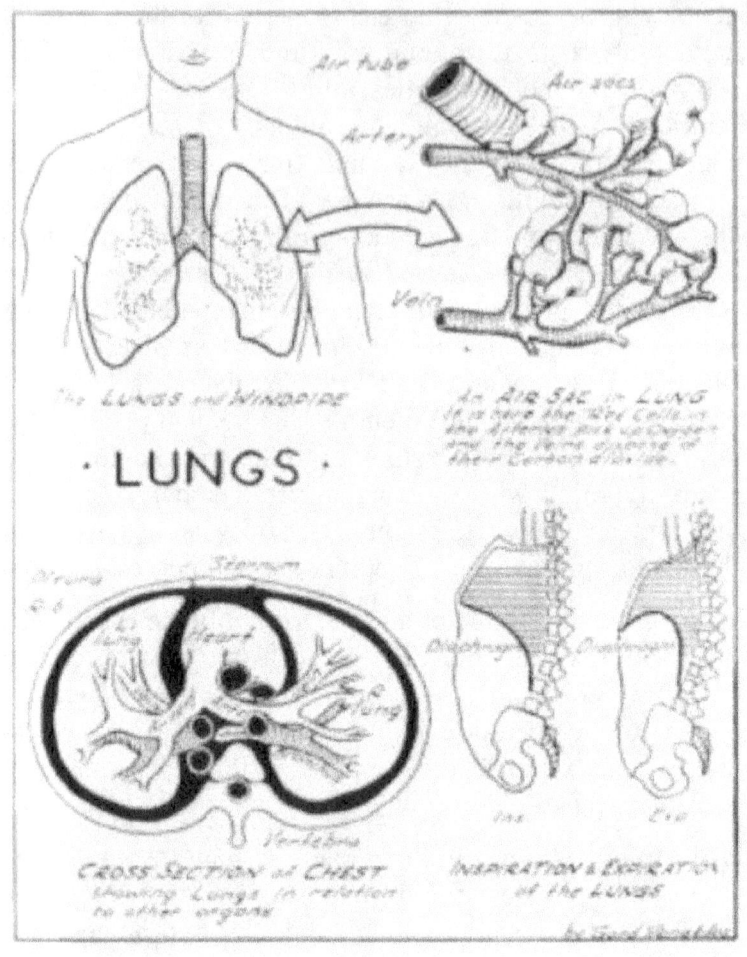

· LUNGS ·

CROSS SECTION of CHEST
showing Lungs in relation
to other organs

INSPIRATION & EXPIRATION
of the LUNGS

Internal respiration also includes two processes: internal oxygen supply or the passage of the oxygen from the blood to the cells of the tissues; internal carbon dioxide elimination or the passing of carbon dioxide from the cells of the tissues to the blood. It is evident that external respiration is a process which takes place in the lungs and internal respiration is a process which takes place in the cells that make up the tissues of the body. The thorax is a closed cavity which contains the lungs. The lungs may be thought of as membranous sacs, the interior of which communicates with

94

the outside air by way of the bronchia, trachea, glottis, etc., while the outside is protected from atmospheric pressure by the walls of the chest.

During life the size of the thoracic cavity is constantly changing with the" respiratory movements. When all the muscles of respiration are at rest, that is at the end of a normal respiration, the size and position of the chest may be regarded as normal. Starting with this normal position, any enlargement constitutes active inspiration, the result of which is to force the air into the lungs. Following this active inspiration, the thoracic cavity may return passively to its normal position, giving a passive expiration, that is, an expiration involving no muscular effort. Normal respiratory movements are of this type, an active inspiration followed by a passive inspiration.

Mechanism of inspiration is the result of the contraction of the muscles of inspiration; passive expiration is due to the elastic recoil of the parts previously stretched. The thoracic cavity is enlarged in all directions—vertical, dorso- ventral, and lateral. The increase in the vertical diameter is brought about by the contraction of the diaphragmatic muscle, which draws the central tendon downward. The dorso- ventral and lateral diameters are increased by the contraction of the intercostals and other muscles which cause the sternum and ribs to move upward and outward. The lungs are expanded exactly in proportion to the expansion of the thorax. As in the heart, the auricular systole, the ventricular systole, and then a pause follow in regular order, so in the lungs the inspiration, the expiration, and then a pause succeed one another.

There is considerable variation in the number of muscles employed in the inspiration, depending upon whether the breathing is quiet or labored. All the muscles which contract simultaneously, including the diaphragm, are classed as inspiratory. Those classed as expiratory contract alter-

95

nately. The external intercostals, levatores costarum, the scaleni, the sternocleidomastoid, the pectorals minor and the serratus posticus superior are the inspiratory muscles. The action of the muscles enumerated is supplemented by additional muscles of the trunk, larynx, pharynx and face, in forced inspirations.

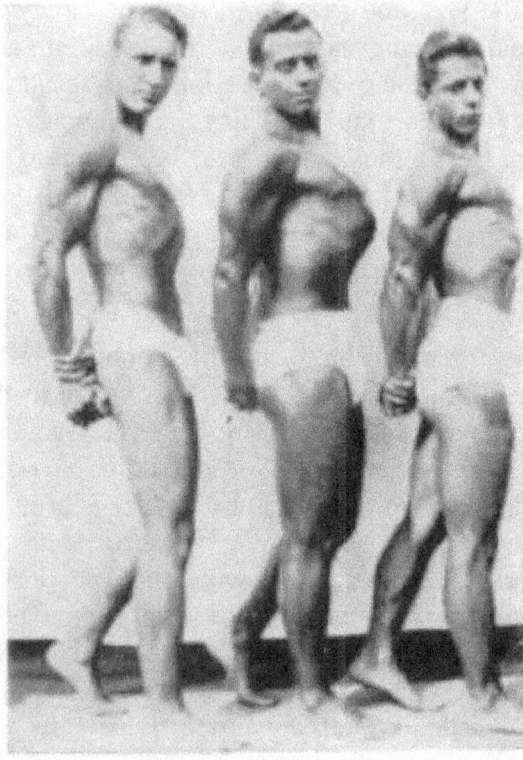

Left to right: Peter Karsavin, for Plaza and Joe Mirasso. Joe was making his start in physical training with weights when Strength and Health magazine was given. He has continued to improve through the years, and in this photo shows a most unusual depth of chest.

It is considered that gravity and the elastic recoil of the lungs cause normal expiration which is usually a passive act. Diminution of the thorax may be caused in two ways in forced expirations: Forcing the diaphragm farther up into the thoracic cavity, a result obtained not by direct action of the diaphragm but by contracting the muscular walls of the abdomen, the external and internal oblique, the rectus and the transversalis, and by depressing the ribs. The muscles which depress the ribs are the internal inter- costals and the triangularis sterni.

It is noted that there are two distinct types of respiration. The sequence of movements is the distinguishing factor. In the costal type the upper ribs move first and the abdomen second. The elevation of the ribs is the more noticeable movement. In the abdominal type, the abdomen bulges outward first, and this is followed by a movement of the thorax. Abdominal respirations are deeper; restriction of the action of the diaphragm by tight clothing is thought to be the cause of costal respiration.

The respiratory center which controls the inspiration and respiration has been described as an automatic center, but sensitive to reflex stimulation of any of the sensory nerves. This brings us to the question of the nature of the automatic stimulus. Experimentally it has been demonstrated that the condition of the gases in the blood has a marked effect upon the activities of the center. The activity is always increased in proportion to the venosity of the blood. On the other hand, the activity is decreased and may fail altogether, if the blood is more arterial than normal. In venous blood the carbon dioxide is increased and the oxygen is decreased. Which of these conditions, the increase in carbon dioxide or the decrease in oxygen, is the more effective stimulus has not been definitely determined. There is much evidence that either factor may act as the stimulus, but the accumulation of carbon dioxide is the more effective.

The average rate of respiration for an adult is about sixteen to eighteen per minute. This rate may be increased by muscular exercise or emotion, in the healthy body. Anything that affects the heartbeat will have a similar effect on the respiration. Age has a definite influence. The average rate during the first year of life is about forty-four to the minute, and at the age of five years about twenty-six per minute. It reduces during the age of fifteen to twenty-five and after that to the normal standard.

The term external respiration is applied to the interchange of gases that takes place in the lungs. Two or three times each minute all the blood of the body passes through the capillaries of the lungs. This means that the time during which any portion of the blood is in a position for respiratory exchange is only a second or two. Yet during this time the following important changes take place: It loses carbon dioxide and moisture, it gains oxygen which combines with the hemoglobin of the red cells and transforms it into oxyhemoglobin, and as a result of this the crimson color shifts to scarlet, and the temperature is slightly reduced.

It is helpful to compare the average amounts of oxygen and carbon dioxide found in the venous blood, and the amounts found in the arterial blood. Average figures for the dog are: Venous blood contains 12% oxygen, 45% carbon dioxide, 1.7% nitrogen. Arterial blood contains 20% oxygen, 38% carbon dioxide and 1.7% nitrogen. In humans the actual amounts of oxygen and carbon dioxide in venous blood vary with the nutritive activity of the tissues, and differ therefore in the various organs according to the state of activity of each organ and the volume of the blood supply. There is always a considerable amount of oxygen in venous blood, also a considerable amount of carbon dioxide in arterial blood. Consequently the main result of the respiratory exchange is to keep the gas content of the arterial blood nearly constant at the figures given. Under normal circumstances it is-not possible to increase appreciably the amount of oxygen absorbed by the blood flowing through the lungs. For the relief of pneumonia, a patient will often absorb unusual supplies of pure oxygen when administered to him which is the result of the oxygen content of the blood of the pneumonia patient being below normal.

The lungs when once they are filled are never completely emptied of air until death. No expiration ever completely empties the alveoli, neither are they ever completely filled. The quantity of air which a person can expel by a forcible expiration, after the deepest inspiration possible, is called the vital capacity, and averages about 3500 to

4000 c.c. for an adult man. Tidal air designates the amount of air that flows in and out of the lungs with each quiet respiratory movement. The average figure for the adult is 500 c.c. Complemental air designates the amount of air that can be breathed in over and above the tidal air by the deepest possible inspiration. It is estimated at about 1600 c.c.

Supplemental air is the amount of air that can be breathed out after expiration by the most forcible expiration. It is equal to about 1600 c.c. Residual air is the amount of air remaining in the lungs after the most powerful expiration. This has been estimated to be about 1000 c.c. Reserve air is the residual air plus the supplemental air in the lungs under conditions of normal breathing, that is about 2600 c.c.

There are other conditions that occur during breathing. However dry the external air may be the expired air is nearly or quite saturated with moisture. An average of about one pint of water is eliminated daily in the breath. On cool mornings this vapor is easily visible. The expired air is nearly as warm as the blood regardless of the temperature of the outside air. A temperature of between 98 and 100 degrees F. is usual. Breathing is one of the subsidiary means by which the temperature and the water content of the body are regulated. The heat required to warm the expired air and vaporize the moisture is taken from the body and represents a daily loss of heat.

The exchange of gases in the tissues constitutes internal respiration and consists of the passage of oxygen from the blood into the lymph and from the lymph into the tissue cells, and the passage of the carbon dioxide from the tissue cells into the lymph and from the lymph into the blood. After the exchange of gases in the lungs, the aerated blood is returned to the heart and distributed to all parts of the body. In passing through the capillaries the blood is brought into exchange with lymph, in which the oxygen pressure is low. The compound of oxygen and hemoglobin, oxyhemoglobin, is only stable in an environment where the oxygen pressure is relatively high. Consequently the blood in passing through the capiilaries gives up much of its oxygen, which passes to the lymph and from there to the tissue cells. On the contrary, the pressure of carbon dioxide is higher in the cells than in the blood, and this facilitates the passing of carbon dioxide from the cells to the lymph, and from the latter to the blood.

It is important to remember that the blood does not give up all its oxygen in the tissues, nor all the carbon dioxide in the lungs. Excessive amounts of carbon dioxide will cause death by asphyxia, but in normal amounts it is as essential to life as oxygen.

As everyone knows the air we need to keep us alive should enter through the nose. Mouth breathing is not normally healthful, for the nose is so designed that it tests the air to see if it is hot or cold, too dry or if it contains dust or other foreign particles. If it is cold it warms it; if too dry it moistens it; if dust-laden it filters it. Incidentally the nose is of paramount aid in making the sounds of talking and of singing. In mouth breathing there is no way to condition the air before it reaches the delicate linings of the lungs.

The function of filtering the air will go on even for two or three days after death. Numerous glands keep the walls of the air passageway moist and thus the dust adheres to them. This lining is called epithelium, and the tiny out- croppings from it which stick out like hairs on a brush, and perform the function of filtering, are known as cilia. They sweep out the dust of the air we breathe and expel it through the nose openings or up into the pharynx.

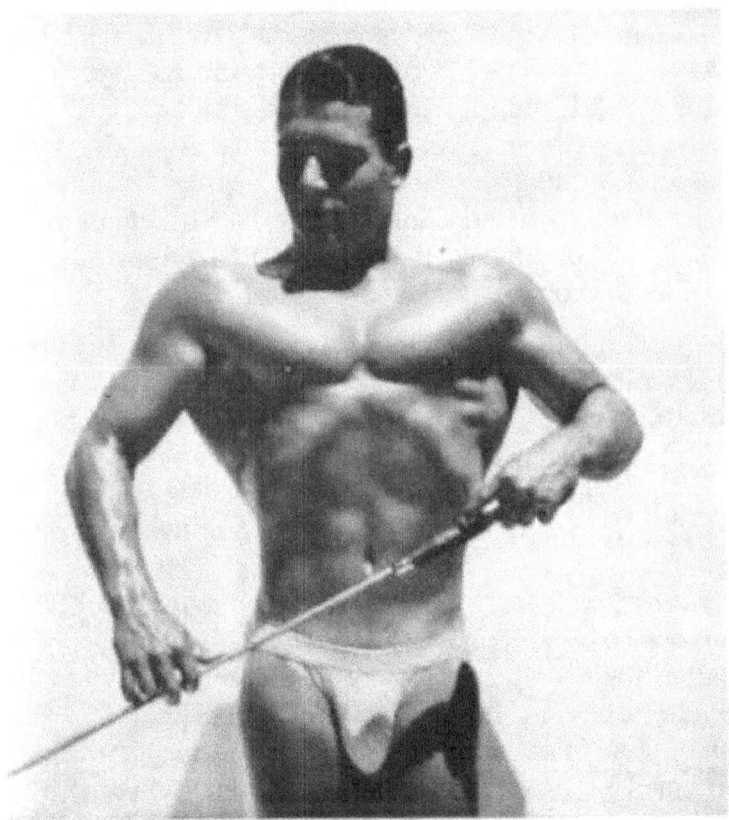

Although we breathe normally seventeen times a minute, when we are quiet or sleeping, respiration will automatically speed up to seventy or eighty times a minute during severe muscular effort when the need for air is great. Breathing is done so automatically, so unconsciously, that few if any of us give the slightest thought to why we breathe or how we breathe. This important and amazingly complicated function is taken for granted. But it's one of the most important phases of operation with this wonderfully made machine of ours, which is our body.

We need air to form combustion which in turn produces motion, heat and chemical products. Every one of the millions of cells in the human body is a tiny engine designed to work somewhat similarly to man-made engines. The engines of our automobiles or factories utilize oxygen and throw off carbon dioxide to produce the motion, heat, electricity, etc., which cause the wheels to turn in factory or with transportation machines such as the truck, pleasure car, locomotive and tractor. Solid fuel formerly in the form of wood, now usually coal, or liquid fuel, oil or gasoline, provides the combustion which produces this power.

Each cell of the body obtains its energy from burning liquid fuel, similar to man-made machines. To do this they must burn oxygen and give off carbon dioxide. The operation of this tiny human engine is so much more complex than that of engines in a factory or in our transportation systems. In a factory and in the case of the locomotive the combustion chamber is separate from the part of the machine which produces the energy. The fire is under the boiler. In automobiles or tractors and in the body cells both combustion chamber and energy-producing parts are combined in one unit. Fire produces heat and light. The slow combustion in the cells of our bodies, while producing a fair amount of heat as in the cells of the muscles and liver, produces other forms of energy too—chemical as in the cells of the glands and electrical as in the cells of the nerves. Light is never produced in the human body, but it is produced in some other forms of life, such as the lightning bug, glowworm, the little deep sea animal with the big name, Noctiluca miliaris.

Each tiny engine in the human body, each of the estimated twenty-five million millions, must be supplied with a regular supply of oxygen and must perform the function of throwing off the carbon dioxide. If the oxygen supply should fail for just one minute, some of the cells are injured and asphyxiated. To keep the body alive it's evident that the supply of oxygen must be constant. In fact, in a reasonably active man, twenty square feet of oxygen is absorbed, transmitted by the blood and used for combustion in a single day. A similar amount in square feet of carbon dioxide is thrown out or excreted from the body. During intensive work a much greater supply of oxygen is required. Unlike some of the smaller animals it is not possible for a human being to absorb oxygen directly from the air through his skin. There is too little surface to supply the body requirements. This problem on which our existence depends has been solved by the action of the lungs. The lungs are an automatic, self-regulating bellows-like organ, which works and continues to perform the same function as long as there is life within us. Presently we will endeavor to explain and describe just how this huge and powerful bellows works. The lungs have mysterious power, in spite of the fact that they are made of soft, spongy, elastic tissue.

The lungs through the function they perform constantly supply the blood cells with oxygen and remove from the blood the waste in the form of carbon dioxide. They are so constructed that they include a surface fifty times as great as that of all the skin on the body. This surface brings in constantly fresh air on one side and with the constantly moving red cells and fluid blood on the other side it makes the exchange of molecules of oxygen for carbon dioxide on the other.

This exchange must take place about three times a minute, more frequently when training or in working intensively. The blood hurrying back and forth has much work to do as it must go through both sets of capillaries to the farthermost points of the body in this normal twenty seconds for a round trip. All of the blood of the body must pass through the lungs, just as it does through the heart and each capillary. The exchange, which takes place in the inner part of the lungs, finds an organ perfectly adapted for this exchange. It is a moist, spongy jelly-like substance designed to dissolve oxygen and carbon dioxide and pass them from one side of the lungs to the other. This vital function, the exchange it is commonly called, which is the essential part of respiration, takes place between the capillaries and the respiratory surface. The remainder of the breathing apparatus merely aids these functions by bringing the fresh air to the respiratory surface and forcing away the used air, rich in carbon dioxide and poor in oxygen. To us breathing is simple, and automatic. It takes place twenty-four hours a day as Jong as there is life within the body. As you must have gathered from this brief discussion, however, the apparently simple process is amazingly complicated when considered more carefully. We will describe the construction of the breathing system, so that you readers who are interested in " what makes us tick " will know more about what takes place within us to maintain or build our strength and our health.

The main part of the lungs is the bellows and it can be seen in the drawing which accompanies this article. It is connected to the outside by a stem, the end of which is the nose; farther along the stem we find the pharynx, the larynx, and the trachea. Man-made bellows have been in use for thousands of years. They have been used since the value of iron or other metals has been discovered.*Ancient or modern, complex or simple, they work in a similar manner, with a valve to let the air in, near the handle, a nozzle to let it out where it can be applied to do the work for which the bellows is designed. This is not practical in the human body; the nozzle is the only opening and through it the air must pass in and out. To further complicate the process the passage of the air must cross the tunnel through which food as it travels from the mouth through the pharynx and the esophagus must pass.

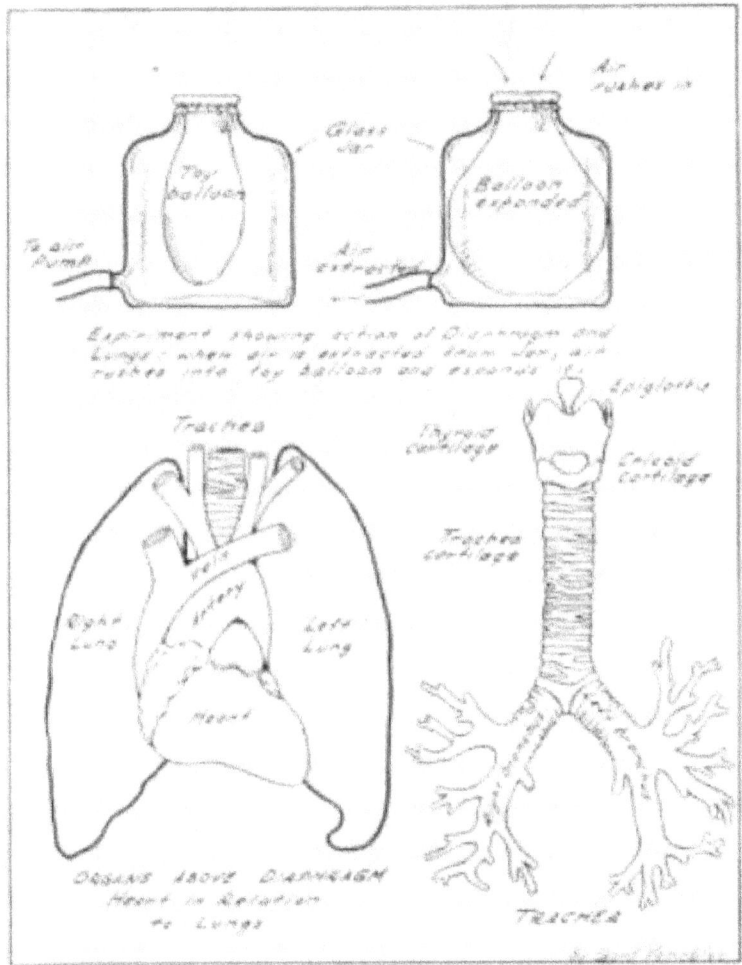

The passage of both air and food is controlled by valves. It's only occasionally that traffic becomes mixed up at these crossings and then you experience the condition of something going down the wrong way. The imaginary green light of the Go system is usually turned on for the air. At brief intervals when food is being consumed, the go sign is turned on for the food and it rushes across as the air is held up momentarily.

The lungs are situated in the cavity of the thorax. You can visualize their position and their function if you imagine a rubber balloon inserted in a bottle. The normal air pressure at or near sea level is fifteen pounds per square inch. Therefore if the air surrounding the balloon is pumped out, air will be drawn in by atmospheric pressure until the sides of the balloon will be pressed out everywhere until they flatten against the sides of the bottle. The action of the lungs in the thorax is similar. A vacuum is created between the thoracic wall and the lungs, so that the outside air pressure is always distending or pressing the lungs against the wall and the lungs by their natural rubber-like elasticity are trying to contract. But the air pressure is always greater than the power of their elasticity, keeping the lungs always distended. It is not far from a balance and very little exertion is required to cause the lungs to function.

In a bellows there are two sides which move toward each other, to draw in and force out the air. In the thoracic cavity of man or all animals higher than the fish, which does not have lungs, an improvement has been made over the bellows because the four sides of the thoracic cavity move in and out. The walls of the cavity change their form with every breath, as they expand and contract. Both sides move in and out; the front wall moves in and out a great deal. There is little movement in the ceiling of the cavity or the back, but the floor moves up and down considerably. The expansion of this cavity sucks in the outside air; its contraction or expiration blows a current of air out.

The sides of the thorax of course are the ribs. Each of these is curved like a bow and to aid expansion they are made flexible through a cartilage which is inserted in the anterior part. The middle of each rib hangs down and when the muscles lift the ribs together, the chest gets wider from side to side. At the same time the breastbone is then lifted up and shoved forward so that the chest becomes deeper from front to back. The outside air pressure forces the lungs to expand, and out against the rib box, so fresh air comes in. If the ribs were made entirely of bone they would break easily, but the cartilages, which have a capacity for twisting somewhat, permit the chest to expand; and yielding as they do to blows or unusual outside pressure in any form, usually prevent the bones from being broken.

It's more difficult for the lungs of humans to work, for with the shoulders not fixed, their weight must be carried by the thorax, and lifted with each movement of breathing. You may have noticed that when a man is out of breath— as after a race or heavy, high repetition deep knee bending — he will lie down or lean over a fence in the former condition, resting his elbows upon the fence. After the deep knee bend in the York courses, the breathing exercise is practiced in the supine position, lying upon a box or bench, which serves the dual purpose of taking the load from the thorax, while enforced breathing is required, but makes possible greater temporary expansion which in time results in a permanent enlargement of the chest. In animals, the canines or quadrupeds who keep their four feet on the ground, the ribs are lifted from the shoulders which are fixed in place. The animals' breathing, you must have noticed, takes place almost entirely from side to side, while in the case of a human being, most of the movement is up and down, a movement of the chest floor which is created by the action and power of the diaphragm. That gives rise to the expression stomach breathing and chest breathing, most persons being comparatively shallow breathers and breathing principally through the diaphragm. Needless to say, any man who trains vigorously, especially with weights, will utilize all the space, all the expansion of his entire rib box or thoracic cavity.

Strengthening Your Heart

ANYTHING that affects the heartbeat will have a similar effect on the respiration. And in this connection we also must remember that anything which affects the breathing also affects the heart as these two organs are partners from the day of your birth until the day of your death. Their operation synchronizes perfectly. When you make demands upon the outer muscles through any form of physical endeavor, particularly of a vigorous nature, there is immediately more carbon dioxide and a greater need for oxygen. The lungs start to fill this demand through increased respiration and the heart keeps pace to make the change which is its work—impregnating the blood with more oxygen and extracting the carbon dioxide, then transporting it through the blood to the place where it is needed.

All authorities agree that the heart is a muscle, and it is a well-known fact that muscles strengthen and improve in their action with use. The body has the faculty to repair itself under almost any circumstances; this is well proven in the case of animals who normally have no doctor—particularly not in the wild state; yet they recover from serious injuries, and overcome the ills which occasionally attack them. Isn't it logical from this brief description to believe that regular exercise with a progressive increasing of the action of the heart and lungs, accompanied by a strengthening of all the muscles inside and out, will also strengthen the muscle which is our heart and improve its action? There is a great deal of proof that hearts have been enlarged and strengthened through regular exercise, that irregularities of construction and operation have been overcome.

But be sure to consult your physician first before launching upon a physical training program, if you have some slight heart difficulty or suspect that you have. The medical authorities report that the heart being only a muscular pump cannot be injured through exercise, but it is reasonable to believe that long-drawn-out or sudden effort, such as in sprinting or the playing of games like football, would not be advantageous for a youth with a weak heart. Gradually stimulating the action of the heart and other organs, through gentle, progressive exercise, has a beneficial effect.

Increased exertion through progressive physical exercise which benefits the lungs also benefits and strengthens the heart. We have heard considerable about enlarged hearts and athletic heart the medical authorities agree that there is no such thing as "athletic heart." There are enlarged hearts, just as there are enlarged biceps or enlarged chests, but larger hearts like larger biceps are stronger and more capable. Nearly one-half of the citizens of this country sever their connections with life through the failure of their hearts. The mortality as a result of heart failure has steadily increased with the years—increased equally as fast as deaths through other diseases have been reduced. Isn't it reasonable to believe that it has come about through the sedentary, indolent lives most moderns live? The hearts of our pioneer ancestors, hard-working men of generations ago, were stronger and more durable than the hearts of the present. Regular exercise will strengthen hearts and should be a source of longer life.

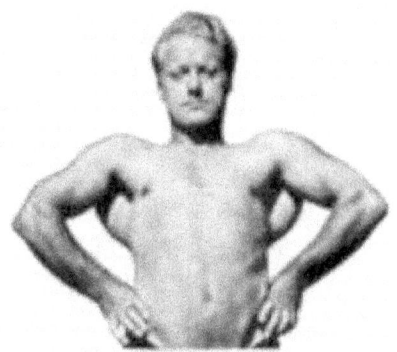

If the lungs are strong the heart will work more steadily; and if the heart is strong the lungs will operate with greater force and evenness. There are many kinds of weak hearts; some are actually defective. The heart may have been weak from[1] birth, although a great many of these so-called weak hearts overcome their own condition. At the age of three I had a severe attack of typhoid fever. Like many children who suffer from such an early severe disease, my life was despaired of. I recovered although I am told the doctor had said I would not live until morning. The report was that I had a weak heart. But a little more than a year later I made it a habit of surpassing the other youngsters in running around a double tennis court across the street from my home. All during earliest childhood I enjoyed what we called " fag '* races—might be more accurately termed fatigue races—the object of the race being to see who could run the longest. Another favorite game was " Buffalo." Our conception of a buffalo herd meant that they went on and on, up hill, down hill, over streams, even over precipices, overcoming all that was before them. We ran all day with our various games and I built such a form of endurance that it was easy enough for me to come home first in a ten- mile modified marathon race for boys under sixteen when I was just ten. Marathons were very popular at that stage of my life and I ran several twenty-six-mile marathons and trained for them regularly. I believe that this regular exercise— chiefly cross-country running—strengthened my heart. Certainly it didn't hurt it, for at the age of forty, when I was examined for a large insurance policy, the examining physician constantly reiterated that he could not understand how a man as large as I, who had been as active and athletic as I, could have such perfect heart action. The blood pressure was right "on the nose" as he phrased it. Yet through my athletic career I had exerted myself to the limit so many times in races that I finished winner, but collapsed at the finish scores of times. I repeat, I believe this great exertion strengthened my heart. Certainly it didn't weaken it. Now modern physicians are convinced that regular exercise strengthens the heart as it does all muscles and other organs of the body.

Hearts should be examined by competent physicians and if the report is unfavorable, certainly that man should not run in a marathon race, row in a four-mile race, or take part in a football game, a long and intensive wrestling match or some similar great physical endeavor. But we must remember that many hearts are weak simply because their owners are weak all over. Their muscles are flabby and covered with fat and it's to be expected that all organs and glands are in the same weakened, sluggish, inefficient condition. If you decide to launch upon a course of physical training and you find that you become greatly fatigued when you walk a half mile, that you pant for breath, and your heart labors when you climb a steep hill, that you quickly become fatigued and breathless when you exercise for a time, you can be sure that your heart and other internal organs are just as weak as the muscles. You can't see the operation of the heart and the other organs, but their - condition definitely manifests itself through the weakness and inefficiency of muscles and fatigue which comes so easily.

A fat man with weak and flaccid muscles may receive the report that he has a weak heart. This is natural, for he is weak all over and with his increased weight he has added many miles of additional capillaries and veins and provided so much more work for the heart to perform. That's the main reason why overweight men are considered to be poor insurance risks. These insurance companies do not take into consideration whether the overweight man has worked enough or exercised sufficiently to have built a strong heart, capable of taking care of a bit of overweight, or whether he is just flabby and soft, and has a heart of similar type. This latter condition is the really dangerous one.

A fat man with a weak muscular heart can easily overtax his weak muscles and it is to be expected that overwork would not be beneficial for his heart, to say the least. But since there is no organic trouble, this man who is out of condition and weak inside and out can by progressive exercise strengthen his heart in conjunction with the lungs just as he can strengthen his back, his arms or his legs through regular and progressive exercise. If such a man will only aspire to attain superhealth, great strength and superb development, there is nothing which will prevent him from attaining that much-to-be-desired physical condition except his own slothfulness or lack of persistence.

How to Develop the Chest

IN my capacity as editor-in-chief of Strength and Health magazine a great many articles concerning the chest are brought to my attention. Many of these advocates of lung culture profess to believe that the development of the lungs is the only way in which a man can hope to become strong, and that practicing inhaling as much air as possible is the only way to enlarge the size of the lungs and ultimately the rib box. With these methods a great many men and boys have attained the ability to inhale from 350 to 400 cubic inches of air and to expand their chests from two to five inches by this internal pressure.

Upon being put to a series of tests the abnormal lung capacity they had developed did not help them in any physical tests. In running a brisk quarter mile it did not prevent them from becoming completely winded and it did not aid them to lift more weight than an average untrained man, who had not spent so much time at expanding his chest. Undoubtedly the practice of constant deep breathing had made them feel better, had given them clearer heads and purer blood, but it had not built power in the muscles, or 120 wind and endurance, as could be proven by running or swimming for a distance.

Many well-known athletes who are stars at their chosen sport were unable to come within a hundred pounds in cubic inch lung capacity of these specialists in deep breathing, but they could lift, run, row or swim for considerable distances. They possessed an effectiveness in performing their normal duty of purifying the blood under enforced pressure which was not possessed by the men who had built increased lung capacity simply through enforced breathing.

This is in line with the fact I offered in a previous chapter that the strongest men have very little actual chest expansion. They do have large-sized, "efficient lungs and powerful heart action—ready, able and willing to perform any task asked of them. Their chests are so near perfection that they are normally held at near their limit of expansion. The chest expansion some tell us about is the result of the ability to greatly expand the muscles which are placed upon the outside of the chest. Muscle control results in much of the phenomenal chest expansion about which we hear. As you can determine by trying it for a moment, it is possible to lift the chest, distend the ribs and pull the diaphragm upwards without inhaling, and a man can also take a really tremendous breath by depressing the diaphragm and without distending the ribs appreciably.

With these thoughts in mind, it would be natural for the uninitiated young man to wonder just what he can do to build his chest. I have mentioned several times that breathing alone, such as by standing in front of an open window in the morning, so favored by physical trainers of another and older day, which is unaccompanied by exercise, has not proven itself to be of much value as a chest developer. When the lungs are not forced to work at an increased tempo as the result of vigorous physical exercise, at a rate well above normal, they cannot be expected to increase in power or endurance.

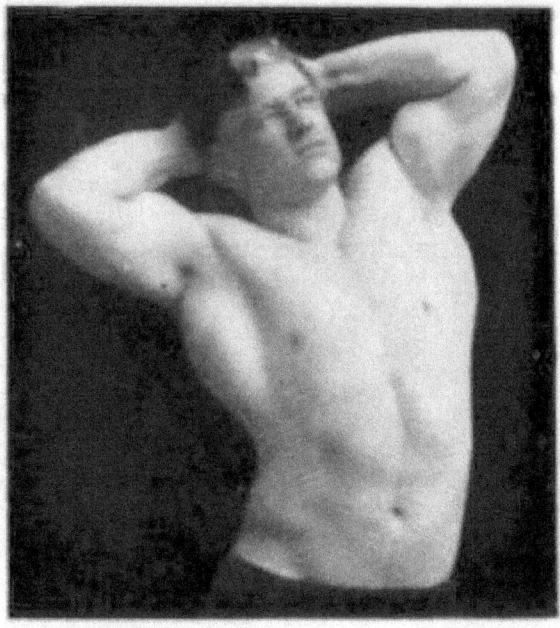

There are two ways to develop the chest: the first, the size of the rib box, the direct result of exercises heavy enough to cause enforced breathing; and the second, the development of the muscles of the chest. Of these the muscles of the upper back will provide the greatest gain in chest measurement. It's surprising how few body builders even consider the muscles of the upper back or the sides when they are striving for increased chest girth. If they think of the muscles at all in relation to greater chest size they think only of the chest, or breast muscles which are scientifically termed pectorals. They spend a large part of their training time developing these muscles, but very little of their time or effort in developing the much larger muscles of the upper back.

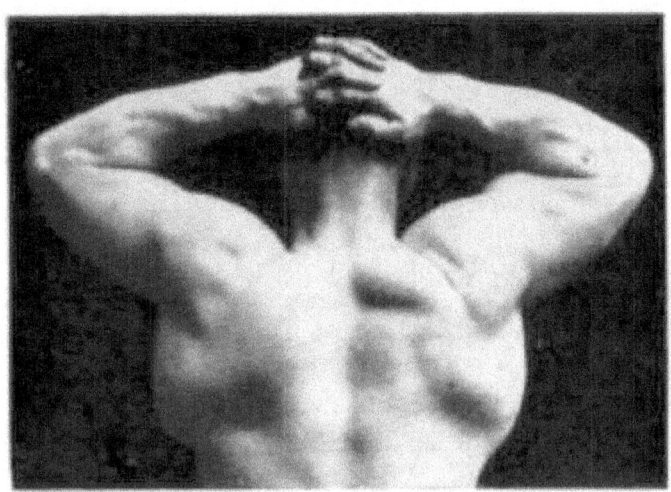

The powerful back and shoulders of Joe Nordquest which made it possible for him to establish a world's record of 388 pounds in the floor press.

Here we have the same condition that is experienced in arm development, as explained in another of my books, " Big Arms." Most men and boys think of just one muscle of the body—that is, the biceps of the arm. The biceps is only about i/iooth of the muscular bulk of the body, yet this muscle receives more attention than any other. The triceps or muscles of the back of the arm are more than twice as large as the biceps, and there are other deep-lying muscles of the arm upon which the ultimate size depends. These seldom seen muscles—the brachialis anticus and the coracobrachial—account for a large part of the bulk of the well-developed arm. To attain the maximum of arm size and strength it is necessary to develop all of these muscles to the fullest extent, yet so many stand in front of the mirror constantly striving to develop their biceps. And with the chest, the easiest-to-see muscles—the pectorals—receive a lion's share of the training time. In the chapter which follows this one I'll offer specific instructions for developing the muscles of the upper back, which will result in the greatest possible increase in chest girth.

It's really surprising that most body culturists think of the chest only as the front part of the body between the armpits. They thus confuse the breast with the chest, while the chest is so much more than just the breast, as it comprises the whole of the torso or trunk of the body from the lowest or floating ribs to well up under the armpits and the clavicles or collarbones. The chest, in other words, is the entire part of the body which is adjacent to the rib box.

In spite of the fact that so many men believe that the chest is just the upper and front part of the body, nevertheless when measuring the chest they pass the tape entirely around them, including within it the sides and back as well as the front or breast. While the measurement they obtain includes the actual size of the rib box, it is greatly amplified by the muscles on the outside of the ribs.

For some reason the usual body builder gives little or no thought to the fact that the muscles of the upper back are included in his chest measurements and that increasing the strength and depth of these muscles will greatly increase the entire chest girth. The accepted method of measuring the chest is to pass the tape entirely around the body with the tape passing across the nipples and around the body under the armpits. Care should be exercised to see that the tape is not held in a slanting position for it is the slanting of the tape which accounts for a good share of the phenomenal measurement of some strength stars.

As the muscles of the upper back are so much larger than those of the front of the chest, being easily twice as large and as deep, as the muscles usually termed the chest muscles, when these huge and powerful muscles are developed to an extent that they become an inch thicker, they account for a full three inches in increased chest girth, according to the geometrical rule that the circumference of a circle is π times the diameter.

Lest you come to the conclusion that your primary training object should be the development of the muscles on the outside of the chest, I want to repeat that increased size of the rib box, with more room or living space for the heart, lungs and other organs, is the most-desired end to strive for. And it's so much easier to obtain a really impressive chest like the greats of the past—Hackenschmidt, Sandow, Arthur Saxon, Louis Cyr, Joe and Adolph Nordquest, Rigoulot or the modern men who are famed for their chest development—Grimek, Stanko, Deutch, Stepenek, Podolak, Peters, Thaler and many others—if you first of all have a big rib box to pack the muscles upon.

We must never lose sight of the fact that the chest and lungs are actually the storehouses of your physical power. Plenty of room for the lungs requires a big rib box, and as we have been constantly stating, big lungs are of tremendous value to any strong man, or to any man for that matter. Big, efficiently-operating lungs enable their owner to continue at intensive work for many minutes, exertion so great that it would exhaust the ordinary individual in a few seconds. This ability may not only come in very handy but be a means of saving one's life under adverse circumstances. I think of one case contained in a story of three fellows who took a vacation in the north woods as spring was approaching. One young man experienced a mishap—broke through the ice—and was carried by the swift current well under the solid ice. There he lay for several minutes, first looking through the ice to see his companions trying to cut through the space, between him and safety—a good foot of thick hard ice. He finally lapsed into unconsciousness but it was possible for one of his companions, Tommy Pedder, former United States junior national weight lifting champion, hailing from Bellville, Ontario, Canada, to swim under the ice and save him. The first man would have died without great lung capacity and strength, the result of bar bell training. Tommy could not have rescued him if he had not had such great lung strength that he could remain for over a minute under the ice bringing out his friend.

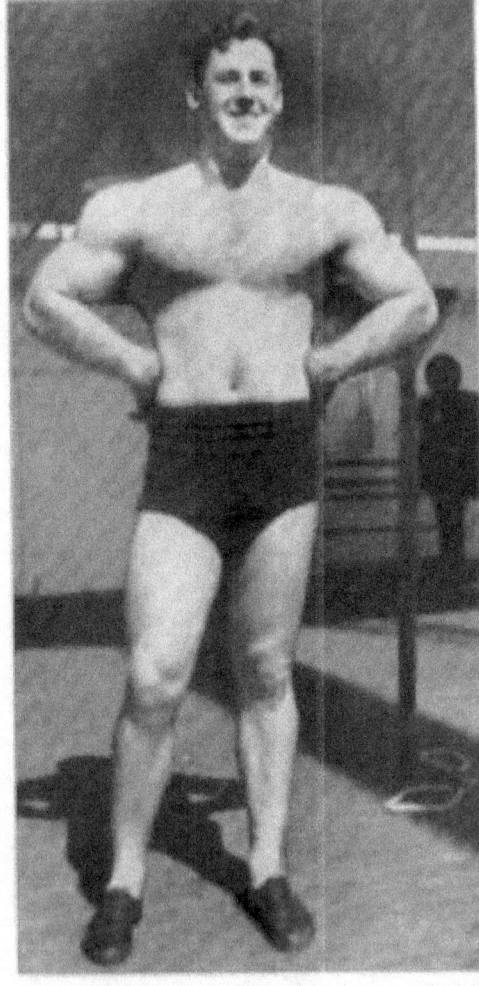

Richard L. Bolster, of the U. S. S. Canopus, of the Asiatic U. S. fleet. He builds and maintains this magnificent body with cable training. Before enlisting in the navy he practiced with bar bells and dumbells.

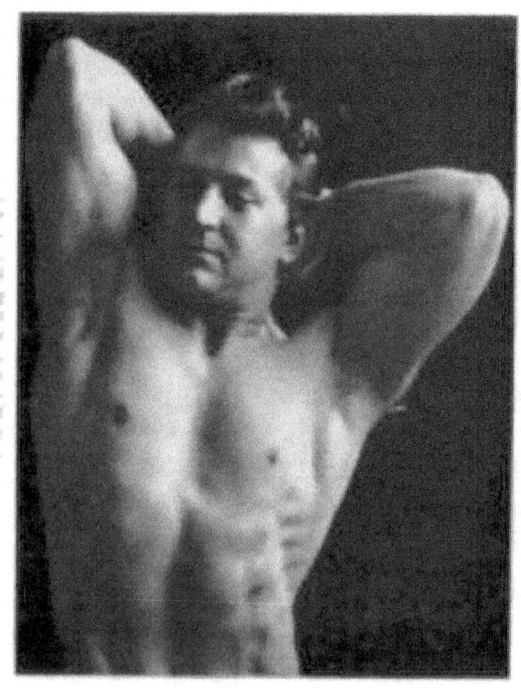

Elmer Farnham, of the York Bar Bell Club. Tri-State Y. M. C. A. 165-pound weight lifting champion, has won many honors for his physique, notably in the national best physique contests and in the York Best Built Man Contest.

Although in the subsequent chapters I am going to launch out in describing the means of developing the muscles on the outside of the rib box, front, back and sides, I don't want you to lose track of what other chapters have contained and to remember that your first aim should be to develop the size of the rib box. And the chief exercises which develop the size of the rib box will not be those which develop the muscles of the upper body. Rather heavy leg and back exercise, coupled with deep breathing, will result in the desired gains in rib box size. Whether you are striving to greatly increase your strength and development, or whether you are just one of the keep-fit enthusiasts, I want to earnestly recommend that you include in your training program many of the exercises which build the chest inside and out.

The practice of these movements for a few months will result in a gain of several inches in your chest girth. It is quite ordinary to gain an inch a month for four or five months, for there are many who have gained as much as three or four inches in a single month's time by the practice of exercises this book contains. And when the rib box grows, you grow all over. There is more space to pack on the muscles of the chest and back, which add to the body weight and the strength; when the rib box is bigger the shoulders will keep pace with it and adjust themselves so that they too will be bigger; but best of all you will find that you feel much better and have far greater endurance with the increased chest size. If you were to practice no additional arm exercises, using the arms little more than as connecting links to hold the weights employed in each exercise—as they are a part of the whole of your body—they increase in size too as your chest grows. Naturally your legs will have grown for they provide much of the effort in the best chest-enlarging exercises.

Some men take up the practice of progressive training with apparatus such as bar bells, dumbells or cables and gain at a phenomenal rate. Invariably these men will possess better-than-average depth of chest to begin. Their organs are in such a position at the beginning that they can do their work well and splendid gains are icgistered. If the beginner has a smaller chest he will not make real gains until his training efforts have resulted in gains of chest size and capacity, so that his internal organs can grow and be in a better position to perform their normal functions. It is so much easier for the man, young or old, who has good chest size, to pack muscles on his body or limbs and thus gain in weight, strength and size.

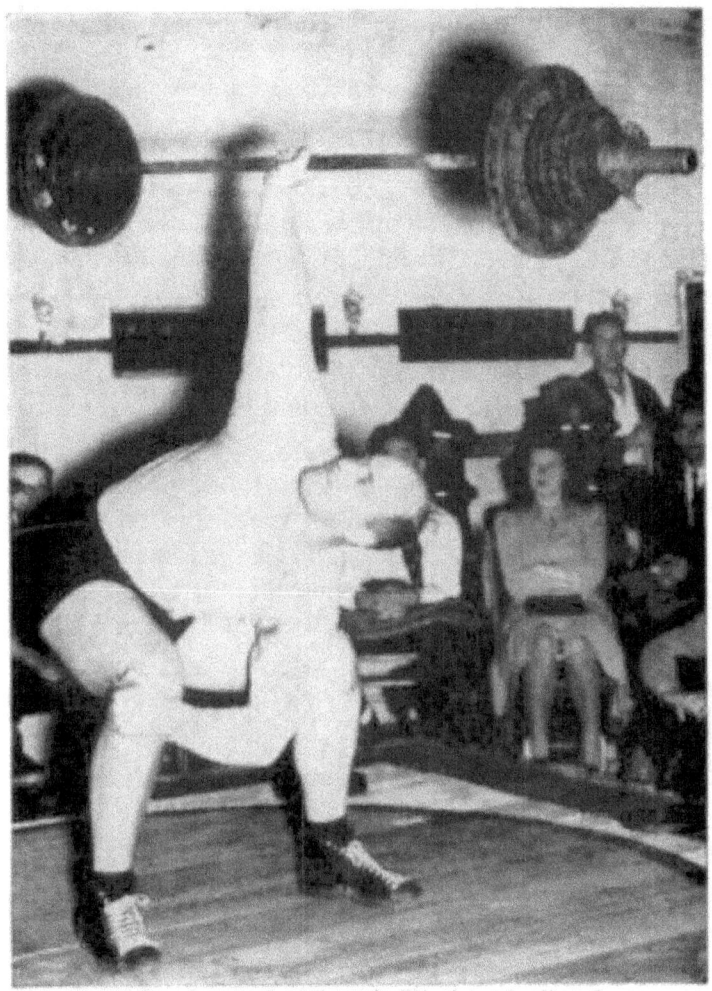

Bob Hoffman bent pressing 275 pounds. This photo taken Xmas Eve at Santa Monica, Cal., in Fanny's Gym, while members of the York team were viewing the action.

The young man who starts out using only dumbells or cables for the upper body will find it quite easy to build muscles on the chest, sides and back, and thus improve his appearance, and while this increased muscular growth will greatly add to the appearance, this man will not be as strong, or as superhealthy, as the man who employs his dumbells and cables so that the big muscles of the legs and back are constantly brought into play, or better still adds a bar bell to his training equipment so that he can make the most of himself physically.

When a man strives not only for muscle building, but most of all for increased rib box size, then things really happen in a physical way. As you will read in the anatomical chapters, the ribs are flexible enough, and so connected to the breast and backbone with cartilages, that they can increase in size even after the age of maturity; remember my own gain of sixteen inches in chest size more than twenty-five years after I reached my present height. And so many others have had similar experiences. A never-ending number of success letters attest to the fact that rib box size can be increased at the age of twenty-five, thirty-five, forty-five or even more. And when the rib box increases in size, we'll say as much as five to eight inches, there will be changes in the adjustment of the other bones. The shoulder blades in some mysterious manner will become set much farther apart, and this great widening of the upper back is not only nice to look at but gives a much greater surface to develop muscles; and of course the muscles add so greatly to the strength. Starting with a very slender, physique, it's most encouraging to see how my own shoulders have widened, and particularly the upper back, about which I will write in the next chapter, has increased.

When the rib box has enlarged and the shoulder blades or scapula have become set farther apart, there is an improvement in leverage, which greatly adds to the power in the upper body. Another statement about my own physical self (kindly pardon so many references to myself, but it seems to me that they are of importance; for when the author of a book using the methods he offers you has obtained the results you want, it's the best proof that he offers you proven methods, don't you think? And lest you think that he might be the exception rather than the rule it is necessary for me to offer you many other concrete examples also)—my shoulders and relative length of arm bones was such that I had a just claim to the not very proud title, " World's Worst Presser." Narrow shoulders, short upper arm and long lower arm gave me an almost impossible-to-overcome handicap that caused me to be such a poor two hands presser that I am the only man in the world to my knowledge who two hands clean and jerked double or more than he could press. Six years ago I pressed 145 and clean and jerked 295. Constant training throughout the years strengthened my body and bettered my physique, broadened my shoulders and set the back muscles farther apart so that I pressed 190 pounds in perfect style, and in almost perfect style 200. Not so much for a big fellow like myself but very encouraging for a man who trained for an entire year before he could press 115 pounds.

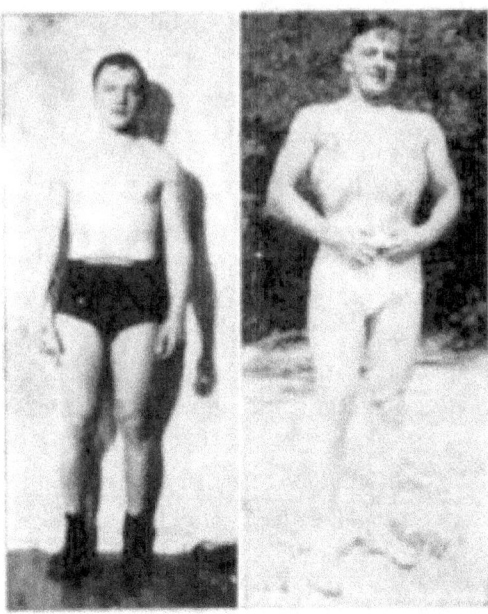

Most weight lifters believe that unfavorable leverage in the two hands press also results in poor leverage in the one hand press commonly known as the bent press method. Yet in this style I have been able to continually improve until my present best of 275 is a modern world's record. Certainly the enlarging of my own chest, the result of the exercises which I am offering with this book, and the adjustments which resulted in much wider shoulders and finally greater strength through more favorable leverage, have resulted in these gains in strength and pressing ability.

It has been my observation, and I am sure that others of experience will agree with me, that a wide-shouldered man with only an average development is stronger than a man with more development and narrower shoulders. Throughout my career I found this to be true to my constant sorrow. It was discouraging to have a sixteen-inch arm years ago and to find men with arms two inches smaller who were stronger than I due to their more favorable leverage. All any of us can do is to make the most of our natural advantages or disadvantages. I did the best I could with mine and would have accomplished much more if I had had more favorable physical features to begin with.

Part of the gain in strength which results from increased chest size is the extra lung capacity, the bigger storehouses of power possessed by the bigger-chested man and part of it is the more favorable leverage which results from the adjustment of other parts caused by this growth of chest. As I go on with the chapters on muscle building, I will include some exercises for the arms and the shoulders which aid in developing the muscles of the chest. This may seem odd at first thought, but not when it is remembered that the deltoids or muscles of the shoulders are involved in all pectoral and most upper back movements. In the majority of big- chested men, the muscles of the shoulders are very well developed and quite strong. From this you can understand that in order to develop the size of the rib box and the muscles which enclose it, exercises which include the deltoids in their action must be a part of the training program.

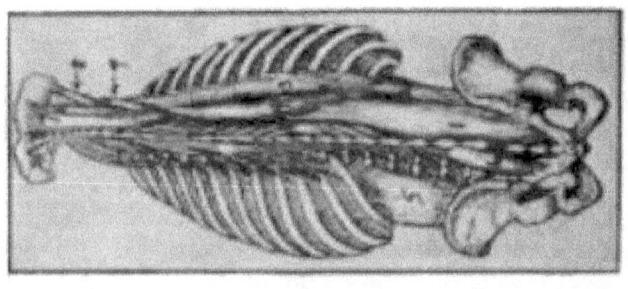

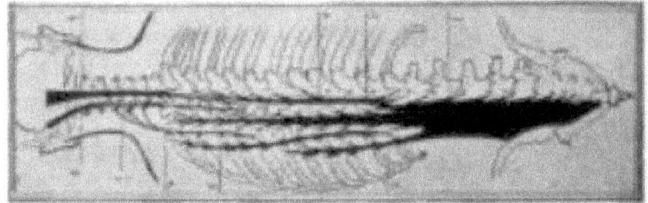

Building the Muscles of the Upper Back

THERE are five layers of muscle on the upper back but only the two larger and outer muscles of these groups are well known to the aspiring body builder. These two are the trapezius and the latissimus dorsi. They form the superficial layer of muscles. The erector spinae is the chief of the deeper lying muscles.

The trapezius muscle, the muscle which is the real badge of the weight lifter or any strong man, imparting as it does the slope to the well-muscled shoulders, received its name because when well developed it forms a diamond-shaped sheet. It has its inception at the occipital bone and extends down to the twelfth thoracic vertebra. Not being familiar with these names you can see from the chart that it extends from well up the neck, across to the shoulders and down at least to the middle of the spine. On the under side the trapezius is connected to the clavicles or collarbone, the acromium process and the spinal column. It is a very large and powerful muscle and completely covers most of the other muscles of the upper back (as well as of the neck and the upper part of the latissimus), particularly the rhomboids major and minor, which will briefly enter into our discussion of the muscles of the upper back.

Its chief function is to raise the shoulders and any weight suspended from them, and only in shoulder shrugging can its great strength really be appreciated. Any advanced weight man can shrug his shoulders while holding four or five hundred pounds in his hands. It is this muscle group more than all others which keeps the shoulder in alignment and this is quite a task when subjected to a heavy load. When Horace Barre set a world's record by carrying 1270 pounds resting on one shoulder across the gymnasium, the strength of his trapezius was the chief force which made this great record possible.

In addition to shrugging the shoulder or carrying weights upon the shoulder, it also will draw the head backward. Here again it demonstrates its great power when advanced strength stars set records of over 500 pounds in the teeth lift. It is assisted by the muscles of the neck and spine but it must perform the greatest share of the work. When only a part of the muscle contracts it draws the neck back toward the side where force is being exerted. The scapulae or shoulder blades are drawn back when the entire muscle contracts, thus bracing the shoulder.

The latissimus dorsi, another muscle group which is the mark of the weight lifter and strong, well-developed man, one that so many strive to develop, imparts the pleasing curve and breadth to the sides of the back. The upper portion of this muscle arises from the lower six thoracic vertebrae well up under the trapezius, and at its lower end it is connected to the three or four lowest ribs and the spine. One of the largest and widest spreading muscle groups in the entire body, the fibres pass in different directions and then converge into a four-sided tendon which is inserted into the lower part of the intertubercular groove of the humerus, or bone of the upper arm.

Its action seems simple enough, for its work is to draw the arm downward, backward and to rotate it. But this can be a difficult task at times, as is evidenced by the size and great strength to which this muscle group is developed in the advanced weight man.

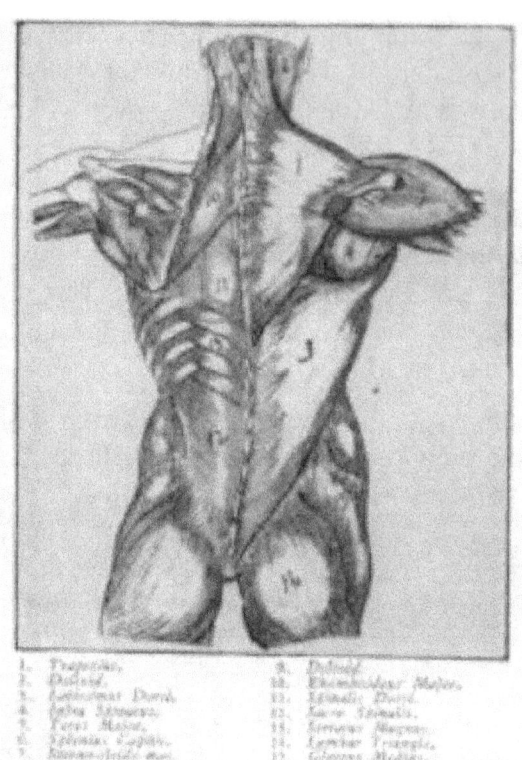

The erector spinae must be included in this study of the muscles of the upper back, as their development is important in adding size to the chest measurement and in performing exercises which develop the entire chest and lungs. It has its beginning at the sacrum and extends to the two lower thoracic vertebrae. As you can easily see from the muscle; chart, it is a solid muscle in the lower back and splits into three columns as it rises. These may be more simply termed than their real Latin names as lateral, intermediate and medial. They are fastened to the ribs and vertebrae at different levels the entire way up the back, extending well up into the neck.

As these muscles climb up the back they establish a goodly number of footholds to assist them in their work. This type of construction is not only continuous but overlapping as one segment begins back of the insertion of the segment below it.

The work of this long and powerful muscle is to maintain the vertebral column in the erect position. With its work to straighten the back, it will do this even against great resistance as when a heavy weight is lifted in dead weight style, or, as in the practice of the competitive lifts when the weight is pulled to the shoulder in preparation for pressing, when it is pulled to the chest in the clean or overhead in the snatch.

In the case of very corpulent men, or with pregnant women, it draws the spine back to counterbalance the forward weight.

In addition to the three major muscles of the upper back there are a certain number of other muscles situated superficially on the trunk which must be included with our study of the upper back muscles. Their chief function is to attach the upper limbs to the trunk and to move the shoulders and arms in any desired or essential way. The chief motivating muscles of arms and shoulders are of course the trapezius and the latissimus (included in this discussion) and the pectorals both major and minor (which will be discussed later).

On the muscle chart you can see some of these muscles which add to the strength and bulk of the upper back and of course to the measurement of the chest. The teres major and the infraspinatus are plainly evident. The rhomboids, rhomboideus major and rhomboideus minor, are visible only when the trapezius is removed. The levator scapulae is also covered with the trapezius and although it will not add to the circumference of the chest it does come into play in practicing most chest-developing exercises and has a position in our discussion. The coracobrachialis, which connects with the arm and also with the scapula, adds some bulk to the chest measurement as do the attachments of the deltoids or shoulder muscles.

The broad and powerful back of champion weight lifter Steve Stanko, showing the muscles which made it possible for him to repeatedly break world's and American records.

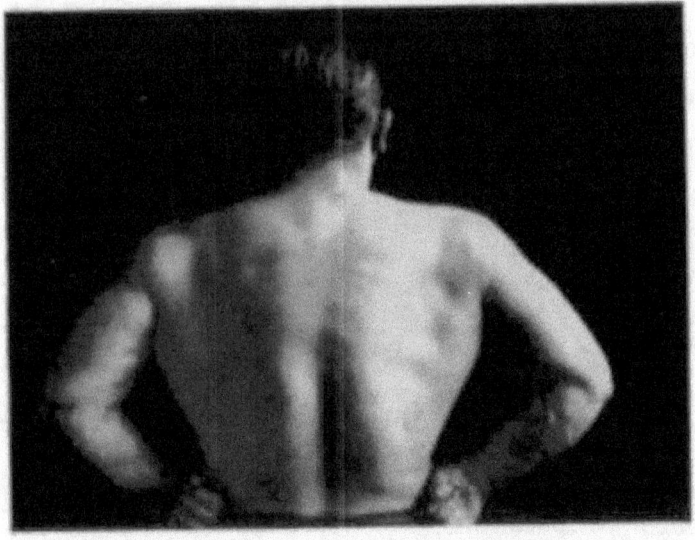

The rhomboids pull the shoulder to the rear. The teres major and minor assist in pulling the arm down, as also does the coracobrachialis. The levator scapulae, as the name implies, raises the shoulder blade; the rhomboids also assist in this movement. The subclavius assists in pulling the shoulder down.

This should be sufficient discussion of the muscles of the upper back, by name and position. If the reader wishes to know more, there are many good books on anatomy which can be had at moderate prices.

This book includes a number of good photos of the upper back, which, in the cases of Fred Rollon and Michael Sulvane, will serve as human anatomical charts. The photo of John Grimek, while possessing muscles so much deeper and less evident than the more finely drawn individual's, gives more than a hint of the development and position of the major back muscles. The common way to show the muscles of the back best is to stand with the upper arms at right angles to the body and the lower arms at right angles to the upper, arm', for this shows the arm, particularly the forearm, to best advantage. The upper back should be spread to make the most pleasing display possible.

The muscles of the upper back can be built easier than any other muscles of the body. Men who launch upon a physical training program show favorable results so much more quickly on the upper back than on the arms or even the legs. I receive so many photos, which would be considered very impressive to the uninitiated, of veritable beginners displaying their back muscles. With this rapid progress and the fact that it is so easy to practice exercises which build the upper back, many men are tempted to spend more than their share of time upon exercising these muscles. There are a great many men like those to whom I referred in the previous paragraph who have gained a reputation as real strong men by showing photos of themselves posed with just the upper back. The experienced body builder, or any man who knows anatomy and the well-developed male physique, could easily see the lack of real development in the upper body and particularly in the legs. While this chapter is devoted to developing the upper back and will contain almost no discussion concerning the development of the lower back, don't lose sight of the fact that from a number of angles developing the lower back is far more important. The developmental effects of lower back exercises will not be as evident as those of the upper back, but a man's vital region is in the lower back, it's the seat of his sexual powers and it gives him strength, spring, power and pep, so don't neglect the lower back entirely in your enthusiasm to develop the more conspicuous muscles of the upper back.

133

We'll start at the top. The trapezius muscles can be seen very clearly in the two photos on pages 145 and 151. In the first photo the shoulder blades are spread and the trapezius is displayed prominently. When the trapezius is flexed it appears as on page 151. We have already discussed the fact that this muscle is shaped like a diamond or an old-fashioned kite, that its chief work is to raise the shoulders or to hold them in place in spite of all the weight that is placed upon them. Therefore the simplest means of developing these muscles is to take a bar bell in both hands with the knuckles front. Your arms serve only as connecting links between the shoulders and trapezius and the weight. They should be permitted to hang as straight as ropes with hooks on the end. While this exercise is simple to perform, the results it produces are little short of astounding.

With each upward movement you raise the shoulders as high as possible, trying to touch the shoulders to the ears as the muscles are raised two to four inches, depending upon your size and the range of your muscles. Harden or tighten the muscles of the middle back by drawing the shoulder blades together. These muscles are extremely powerful and can be subjected to very vigorous work.

All weight lifting movements are highly beneficial. In fact weight lifting is the only way in which these muscles can be developed to their limit. All advanced weight lifters can display these muscles in an astounding way. Their constant practice of the three lifts, when heavy poundages are reached, are sufficient to develop the muscles to their limit.

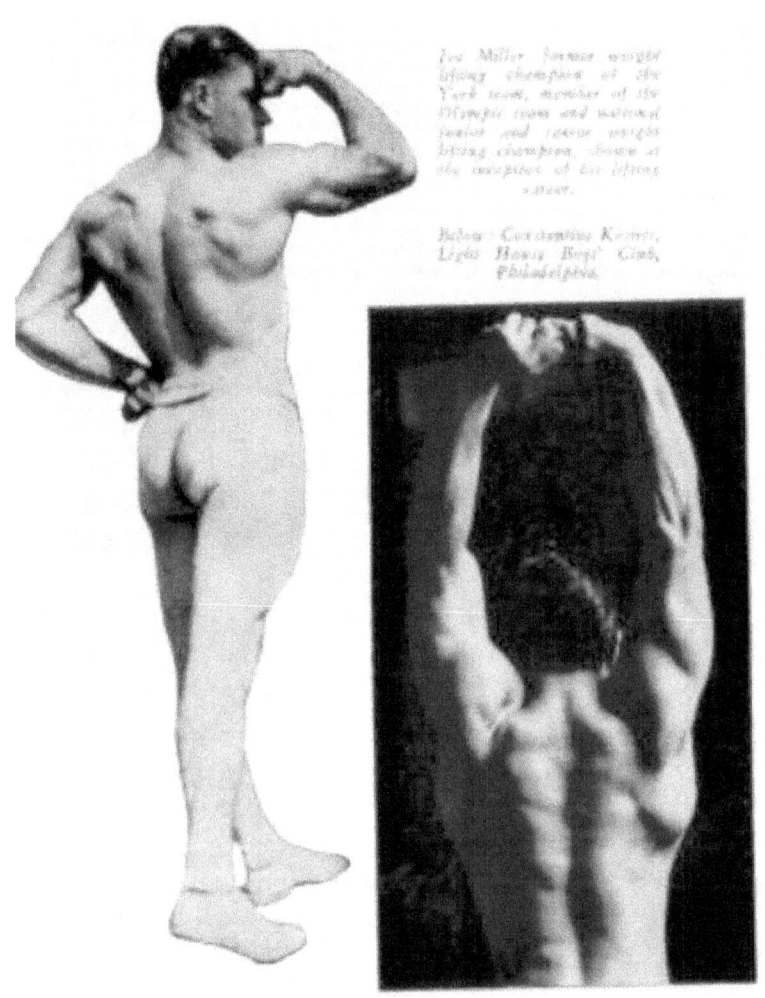

In pulling weights to the shoulders or overhead, the trapezius group, assisted of course by the legs, back and arms, are the chief motivating force. Men like Grimek and Stanko, so often mentioned in my books, have tremendous development of these muscles. When the arms are flexed and the shoulder blades drawn in somewhat, a round deep depression which would hold a full pint of milk is evident. These men not only practice very heavy single attempts as in competitive lifting (Stanko has records of 310 and 390 in the snatch and clean and jerk respectively), but they practice a great deal of lifting exercises. Stanko will perform five or six repetitions with 260 in the two hands snatch and several with 350 or more in the two hands clean and jerk.

In single attempts as well as repetitions, they strive to obtain all the pull they can and if you will closely examine the action pictures of leading lifters which appear in the book "Weight Lifting," you will see that the shoulders are pulled high and the trapezius is under tension as in performing a shoulder shrug. Practicing repetitions in various ways in the three lifts, from the stiff-legged position, with the back only, starting slowly and finishing fast with a strong second pull and lift of the shoulders, will produce splendid results in building these muscles.

The three lifts—two hands press, snatch and jerk—are the chief lifts which are practiced today, but all lifting is highly beneficial in the developing of these muscles of the back, shoulders and of course the spine. Two other quick lifts, formerly a part of the official lifting program—the one hand clean and jerk and the one hand snatch—are good trapezius developers. Repetitions with the one hand snatch will develop chiefly one side at a time, so exercise both arms successively. The one arm swing is another good lift to practice.

Very heavy lifting such as the straddle lift, or the seldom practiced hand and thigh lift, provides excellent work for the trapezius. Over a thousand pounds can be handled by a strong man in this manner. Five or six hundred in the straddle lift can be utilized, while even the smaller men make repetitions with four hundred pounds. A strong man could fasten his hand to a bar bell, aiding the grip by means of a handkerchief or other cloth, lift the weight first as a one hand dead weight lift, and then raise it inches more just by shrugging one shoulder, even if the bar bell weighed four

hundred pounds. I have seen such a feat of strength performed. Lou Schell" a member of the original York team,
who still lifts occasionally and is most famed for being the
father of fifteen children (no multiple births) by the time he
was thirty-two, weighs only one hundred and thirty-five,
but can perform this feat with three hundred and fifty
pounds.

Experts at muscle control can execute the most astounding
feats in moving the shoulder blades, which of course is
done by the trapezius muscles.

As the trapezius is designed to lift the shoulders, all exercises which cause the shoulders to be raised under the
resistance of weights or cables are beneficial. An
alternative way to practice the usual shoulder shrug is to
pull the weight as high as possible, bend the shoulders far
to the rear while keeping them high, then lower them while
holding the shoulders back, raise again, move the shoulders
forward, and continue with this movement until tired. It
should be possible to perform trapezius movements at least
twenty repetitions.

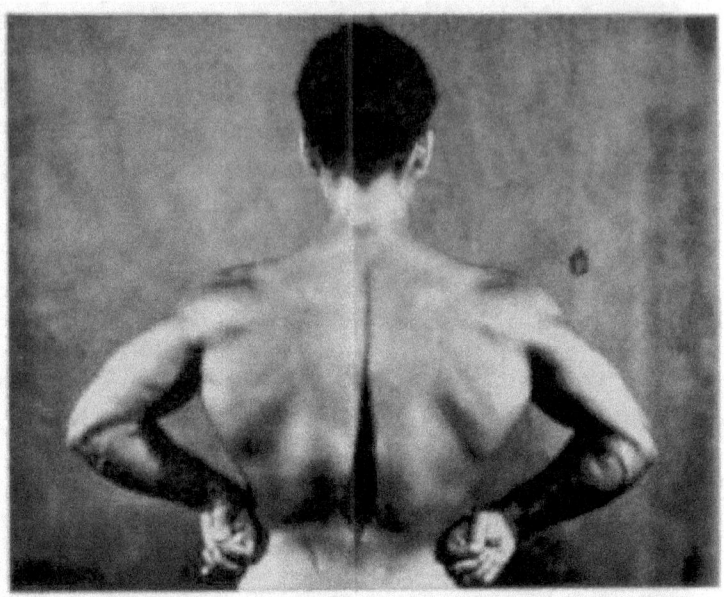

Tom Carter, 18 years of age, displaying as fine a back as one could hope to see. Note particularly the slope of the trapezius, the broad curve of the latissimus and the depth of the same spinalis.

Dumbells permit a greater range of movement than bar bells but they cannot be loaded quite as heavily. With dumbells, shoulder elevating can be practiced alternately, and a much greater range of rotation in conjunction with shoulder raising is possible. With cables, the two arm press with the cables behind the back is a good developer for the trapezius, particularly when you bring the shoulder blades in as far as possible and expand the back as far as you can with the alternate movement. Employing the stirrups, the shoulder shrug and upright rowing motion are good exercises for this important muscle. One of my favorite exercises is the upright rowing motion with dumbells. Pull the dumbells from a position in front of -the thighs with the knuckles front until they are chin high, the shoulders raised and the bent arms held out to the side.

Most body-building exercises involve the trapezius in some manner and it will obtain a fair share of development without specialization of any sort. For the trapezius and most of the other muscles in the body, particularly the upper body, are brought into play with nearly every exercise. Chinning, dipping, rowing motion with bar bells, dumbells or cables (particularly when the shoulders are drawn well back at the completion of the movement), all the lifts, hand balancing, understanding in pyramid building, rope climbing, wrestling, in short any good exercise, will have some beneficial effect in developing the trapezius as well as other muscles of the upper body.

Prior to the advent of the various courses which I offer to the strength and development seeking public, there were courses which informed the world that a man could obtain all the strength and muscle he wished by practicing a few key exercises. Frequently they offered a man as exhibit A, who had exercised primarily with a few well-known exercises such as the dead lift, deep knee bend, and the two hands press—all good exercises. There are an estimated number of four billion muscular fibres in the body, all planned to assist in moving some part of the body against resistance of some sort—720 muscles, designed to move the body in every conceivable and diverse manner—so the practice of many exercises is essential.

We are born with all the muscular fibres we will ever have, and the difference between the immature frame of the slender, undeveloped young fellow and the powerful, beautifully built body of John Grimek is simply the strengthening and enlargement of these muscular fibres through movements which bring as many of the 720 muscles as possible into play. So isn't it logical to believe, as we do, that best results are had with the practice of a wide variety of exercises? I usually term it the "1000 exercises."

It's been definitely proven that men who practice a few exercises, using and developing the muscles in the same groove always, will not become as strong as the man who

139

practices many diverse movements. A combination of heavy lifting, with lifting motion exercises and many body-build- ing exercises, has built the magnificent bodies, great strength and athletic ability of the York Bar Bell Club champions who hold all the United States records in the Olympic body weights and three fifts and totals, most of the world's records, and all of this year's official national championships.

If you were to delve into the life and training of any well-built man whose friends claim that his physique is the result of the practice of only twelve or fourteen good bar bell exercises, you would learn many things. You would certainly find that he was a skilled hand balancer (practically all exceptionally well-built men are); very likely he is the understander in practicing hand to hand work, and the understander in pyramid building at the beach. At times he shows his ability with the cables and exceptional ability at strand pulling comes only from practice. In his home gym he has a chinning bar and, quite likely at least, a pair of two by fours to practice dipping, as with a parallel bar. He has a rope for rope climbing, and quite a bit of special apparatus to improve his grip and forearm strength, even a teeth lifting outfit, a hip lifting belt and plenty of weights to use with it. It is quite likely you will find that he practices tumbling and has done considerable wrestling. Although it is claimed that he " body builds " only with bar bells, his friends will enthuse over the way he pulls up heavy weights in the snatches and cleans and the way he jerks the latter overhead.

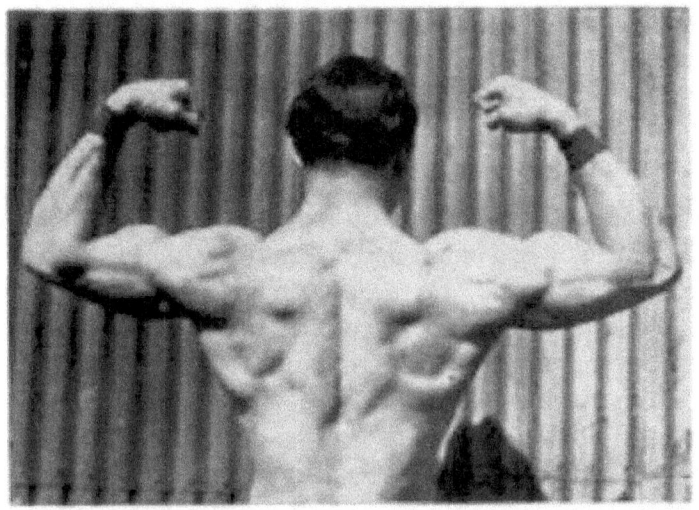

Kenneth Terril, one of the men most famed for his physique a generation ago. For long he was a professional vaudeville performer. He built
the foundation for this fine physique through cable stretching.

This reminds me of a man who has been one of the heaviest
advertisers of his physical culture course for many years.
He claims to have built his formerly splendid physique
through his own system of exercises to which the name "
Dynamic " has been applied in various manners. He denies
that he has followed other forms of exercise, yet when we
brought a great deal of proof, many witnesses who knew
how he trained, he stated under oath that he did not train
with weights—he only used them to demonstrate his
strength. Three times a week at least, sometimes four, he
demonstrated his strength with weights and cables. But the
story of his life and training which brought his physique to
the point where it was selected as the best built in America
in 1920, although the best-built men were not in the contest,
tells us that he trained with bar bells and cables. He spent
years demonstrating cables in sporting goods stores
throughout the east, he became good enough at hand balancing, tumbling and strength feats to spend some time on
the stage with a partner, he became a fair wrestler and did a

lot of swimming and really heavy lifting to demonstrate his strength. He claimed a 270-pound bent press, and you fellows who have tried this lift certainly know that years of weight training practice was necessary to learn the form and to acquire the strength to hoist such a great poundage.

The few illustrations I am offering point to just one fact: Although there are some best exercises to build the shoulders, the upper back, the pectoral muscles, to internally increase the expansion of the chest, the practice of a great many exercises—the thousand exercises—is invariably responsible for the development possessed by the leading men of might and muscle. Men like Klein, Sansone, Asnis, Deutch, Schusterich, Thaler, and our own York champions as well as countless others, well known throughout the world for their strength and symmetrical bodies, are the products of all-around training. Every one of these famous strength athletes has trained with the knowledge that strength and well-developed roundness of all the muscles is the result of practicing a great variety of exercises.

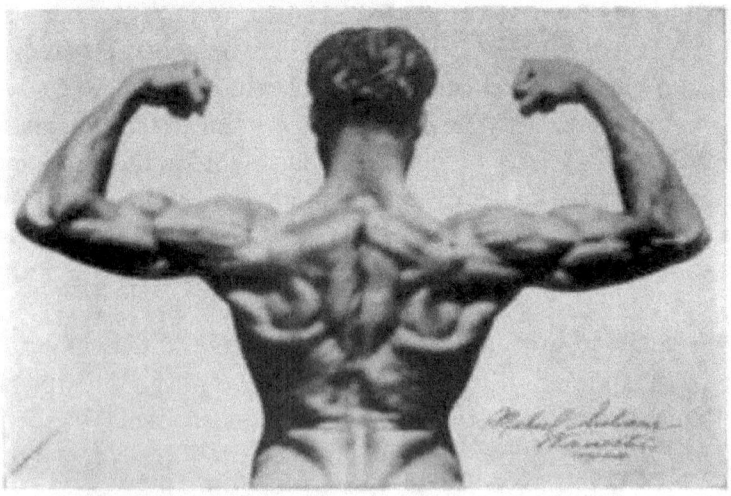

The back of Michael Salvoms, a human anatomical chart, which shows most of the muscles of the back to good advantage.

Developing the Latissimus Dorsi

IF you examine closely the backs of the best lifters and the best weight-trained men, particularly those who use cables in their training, you will note that the waist is apparently narrower just under the floating ribs, and from that point to the armpits there is a powerful muscular curve. This curve results from the development of the biggest muscles of the back, known as the latissimus dorsi. As we briefly mentioned previously their main function is to pull the arm downward and backward and to rotate the arm inward.

If you were to visit the York Bar Bell Gym you would be impressed with the fact that all of our champions look broader across the back than they do in the front. This is the result of well-developed and powerful upper backs, par-ticularly the development of the latissimus. These weight lifting stars have practiced the exercises which I am offering in this chapter although their near-perfect all-around development is chiefly the result of practicing repetition weight lifting exercises. If you apply yourself in a similar manner, you too will broaden your upper back and obtain the breadth and curves which are the mark of the superbly built, really powerful man.

Few of us have the opportunity to practice Roman ring exercises which are really the best for developing the latis-simus. While such exercises would not be possible for a heavy man, the man of average size who can draw himself up on the rings, the arms straight and extended to the side, is sure to have most excellent latissimus dorsi development. The best exercises we can devise are those which permit the progressive practice of exercises similar to those which are practiced on Roman rings. On the Roman rings a man must start with body weight. With exercises practiced with cables and overhead pulleys, a very slight resistance can be used in the beginning, and from that point by gradual in-creases, as little as one and a quarter pounds with weights or one strand with cables, progress and increases in strength and development of the muscles under discussion can be attained.

But don't form the impression that, because these muscles are developed by pulling the arms down, they cannot be developed by weight lifting. At first thought it would seem that only muscles which will benefit from putting weights overhead will be developed, that the strong force of gravity will bring the weight down unassisted, but the muscles which pull down as in Roman ring work, chinning, rope climbing, or cable pulling, are brought into vigorous action in practicing the two arm pull over. As I will later state, this best of all chest-developing exercises, the two arm pull over, should be practiced with straight arms to bring maximum benefit in internally expanding the chest or developing the pectoral muscles. But to bring maximum results in latissimus development a very heavy weight should be employed and the arms may be bent as the weight is drawn over the face. It is evident from this discussion that pulling the weight over in preparation for a floor press, usually termed the supine press, will have a splendid effect in developing the latissimus muscles.

In the room where I am writing this chapter is a number of photos chiefly of our team at various times. Right before my eyes is a photo of the team I sent to Paris for the world's championships in 1937. Tony Terlazzo and Johnny Terpak came back with the world's titles in their respective classes. Tony has long presented from the back what I often call a professional appearance, with his powerful and broad back and exceptional curve of the latissimus. Gord Venables, the next man in the photo, has a really splendid sweep to his latissimus. No doubt some of this fine spread was originally developed through swimming, as he was back stroke swimming champion of Canada some years ago; he can swim back stroke as fast as most good swimmers can propel themselves through the water with the crawl stroke. The third figure from c left is Dick Bach- tell, the 132-pound champion in nine years and a place winner on other occasions. Weight lifting and gymnastics, including balancing and tumbling at which he excels, built the breadth of his back. Next to him is Johnny Terpak, the world's best middleweight lifter. His great back is chiefly the result of weight lifting exercises—practice of the quick lifts at which he is phenomenal. He holds all the middle-weight records in his class.

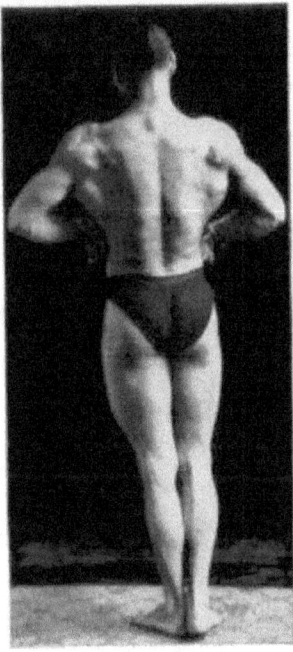

But the center figure is the one which is most interesting in our present discussion. For in the center of this group is the national heavyweight champion of 1937, 265-pound Dave Mayor. Dave made his start in life as a four and a half pound baby. He grew to young manhood and his present height of a bit over six feet, weighing 120 pounds. From that point in a few years' training, most of it performed in his mother's kitchen, he built a 265-pound body and was America's strongest man before he entered professional wrestling. He is best known as the possessor of 19 - inch arms which are the largest muscular arms in the world. You will observe another feature which has seldom been mentioned, concerning Mayor's development—tremendous breadth and depth of the muscles of the upper body. As Dave never performed side or abdominal exercises, and could eat " like a horse," he is carrying some surplus weight around the waist. This detracts somewhat from the wedge-shaped appearance he would otherwise have possessed, but it cannot entirely eliminate the very exceptional width and curve to the latissimus.

Dave's favorite exercise is the rowing motion when holding the body in the bent over position. His ability in this exercise was almost unbelievable and most of the fame he won, the honors he garnered, and the physique he built, came through the practice of this exercise. In his lifting, at which he established United States records in the two hands press, two hands snatch and two hands clean and jerk, he did most of his lifting with his arms, upper back and shoulders. Had he been able to employ more fully the really powerful muscles of the legs, it would have taken years for John Davis, who holds the present world's and U. S. records in the heavyweight division, or Steve Stanko or Louis Abele, to have surpassed these records.

It is easy enough to row with 100 pounds, that is, easy enough for any advanced weight-trained man and if you can row with 150 pounds correctly, without a lot of back movement to supplement the strength of the arms and muscles of the upper back, you can consider yourself to be very strong. The rowing motion at one time was a favorite of mine and I have performed ten correct rowing movements with 180 pounds, while my forehead rested upon the back of a chair to insure little or no back movement. But Big

146

Dave has done this with 200 pounds, ten repetitions. And with fast movement and some body action he has frequently practiced this splendid movement with 300 pounds. You can obtain a fair idea of the great strength of Dave Mayor's latissimus by comparing your own record with that of his in rowing.

Rowing may be practiced in a variety of ways; with the bar bell several methods are possible. The usual manner of rowing is to pull the bar to the chest with the grip of the hands more than shoulder width apart, keeping the elbows far out from the body as the weight is brought to the chest. A closer grip, pulling up the weight with the elbows close to the body, will provide a somewhat different range of action for the muscles. Normally the bar touches the chest near the shoulders but at times you should touch the body with the bar low upon your chest or even upon your abdomen.

Another little known and splendid result-producing form of rowing is to lie face down on a rather high bench or a heavy plank placed across two carpenter's horses, boxes or platforms of some sort. Pull the weight up until it touches the board just below the chest in the first style of practicing this special method. This has the advantage that the body is supported, and that there is no opportunity to supplement the movement by aid from the back. The upper back, particularly, and the arms exert the full force in this movement and receive the chief benefit.

This same position makes it possible to practice another good latissimus developer. Keeping the arms straight, raise the weight to a position just below the thighs. You'll feel the muscles which result from the practice of this exercise after you have made a number of repetitions.

Before going on with additional exercises I wish to digress for a moment. While counting the number of movements with each exercise makes it possible for you to definitely measure the amount of work you are doing, the actual counting prevents you to some extent from concentrating fully on the correct performance of the exercise which you are performing. If you will contract the habit of continuing each movement until comfortably tired, concentrating the full force of your mind upon the muscle group involved in the exercise, superior results will be attained. While it is necessary to really extend yourself at times, to make stern demands upon the muscles, to work on your nerve, to work up to or beyond your best efforts of the past, you should never work on your nerve more than once a week. On the usual training night you should continue with a movement until you are comfortably tired. Don't confuse laziness with being really tired, but continue with the movement you are practicing at the moment, for a count or two after you feel the exercise considerably.

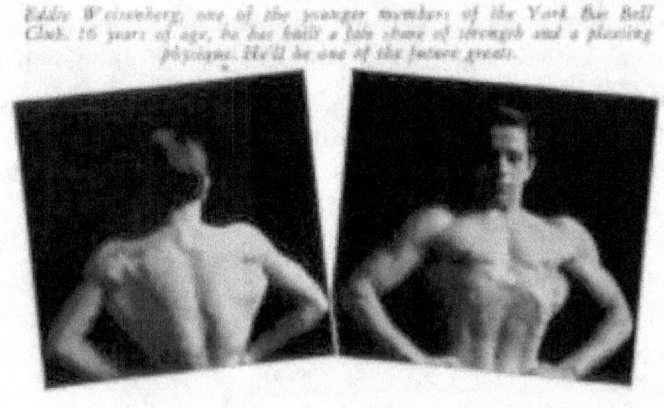

Eddie Weinberg, one of the younger members of the York Bar Bell Club. 16 years of age, he has built a fine share of strength and a pleasing physique. He'll be one of the future greats.

When more than half body weight is employed in the rowing motion some effort is required to keep the body balanced and from toppling forward. Rowing with a bar bell does not give the upper back muscles the full range of movement, as the deeper your chest, the sooner the bar touches it. Therefore single and alternate arm rowing with

148

dumbells should be a part of your training program. Leaning forward and alternately rowing with a pair of fifty-pound weights, or even seventy-fives or more for the stronger, heavier men, dropping the weight to the lowest possible point and pulling it very high will produce splendid results. But the one arm rowing motion with the body leaning over and the other hand resting upon a low box is one which permits the greatest range of action. As the chair or low box braces your body you can put much greater effort into the rowing motion and pull so much higher. Your ability in this form of rowing will rapidly increase and soon you will find yourself able to row single armed with seventy- five to one hundred pounds and, best of all, you will have made a great improvement in the thickness and shape of the muscles of the upper back.

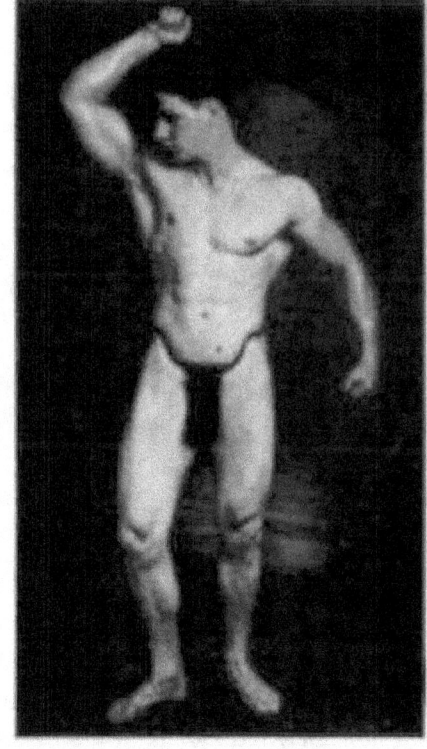

Jack Channing, of the Pittsburgh Central Y. M. C. A., another fine shows York Bar Bell man. While not a competitive lifter, his records in the three lifts are very commendable. He has been winner in national best built man contests.

There are a number of dumbell exercises which are of importance in developing the muscles of the upper back. One of the best of these is to lean forward with the upper body at right angles to the legs; keeping the arms straight, swing dumbells to the side and at shoulder height, lowering them until they are suspended below the body. This is a splendid developer of the upper back. A few years ago I had a visit from a well-known strong man who told me that this was his favorite exercise. One morning while I was shaving and we were at our summer bungalow, I looked out the window and counted twenty-two repetitions which he made in this exercise while utilizing a pair of forty-five-pound dumbells. One of this man's favorite positions was to lie upon the floor while reading, chest down, legs straight, feet turned to the side as a Polar bear frequently lies, with his upper body propped up on his elbows. In this position the development of his trapezius and upper back muscles showed their truly imposing proportions. Another good dumbell exercise, primarily used as a developer of the triceps, is to lean forward, holding the dumbells at the sides with the upper arms parallel to the body; extend the arms backward, straightening them and at the same time hardening the latissimus. All forward and lateral raises, while numbered among the best developers of the deltoids, also bring the trapezius and the latissimus into action. There are so many good dumbell exercises which aid in the development of the upper back. The only objection to dumbell training could be that they don't provide the heavy resistance that can be had with bar bells, so very heavy work with bar bells must occupy a major portion of your training time.

We must remember that practically all lifting movements involve the muscles of the upper back to a considerable degree. In practically any exercise where the bar ball is lifted to the chest, the upper back is bound to be heavily involved. The phenomenal backs of the great old time strong men—

Saxon, Cyr, Sandow, Rolandow, Gorner, Cyclops, Rigoulot, Barre—and equally famous but still living greats— Travis, Davis, Abele, Grimek, Stanko, Steinborn, and Klein—all illustrate the wonderful backs which will result from pure lifting.

Most of these men are stars at very heavy lifting. Gorner and Rigoulot, in particular, were exceptional at dead weight lifting, Travis and Cyr at harness and platform lifting, Steinborn and Rigoulot at the quick lifts, one and two hands snatching, and one and two hands cleaning and jerking. Sandow and Saxon were particular stars at the bent press. They trained hard with the sole intention of establishing records, but they built great physiques, particularly excelling in the muscles which we are discussing in this part of the present volume.

In any form of lifting from the floor and standing erect with the weight, the upper as well as the lower back is directly involved. In overhead lifting the arms must be drawn back as they are straightened. In cleaning and snatching, although leading lifters endeavor to pull the weight straight up, the bar in the snatch is thrown back as the wrists turn and pulled well in at the shoulders for the clean. Much of this strength is imparted by the latissimus muscles. In the dead weight lift if the shoulders are brought well back as they should be, as best results are attained by exercising the muscles over the greatest possible range (from extreme of extension to extreme of contraction), the latissimus and the trapezius will obtain maximum benefits from the movement.

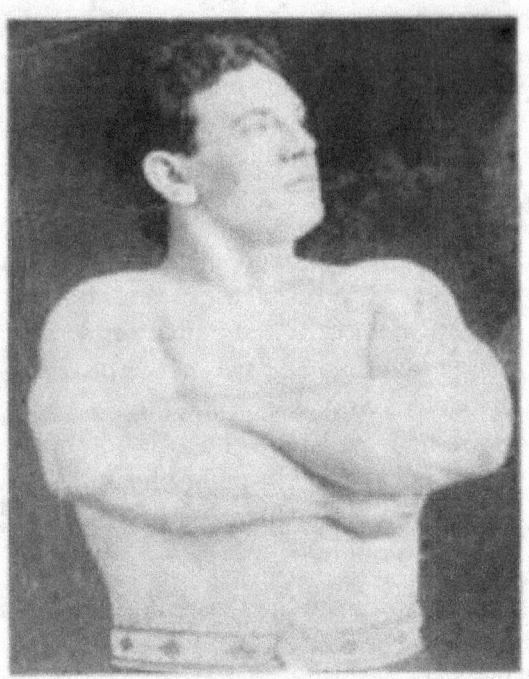

The bent press is a great developer of the latissimus. A heavy bent press creates terrific pressure and contraction of the muscles on the side of the body. The shoulder blades are pressed tightly together midway through the lift, are separated as the arm is straightened and utilized in a different manner as the weight is held overhead. Supporting the tremendous weights which are possible in this position will develop the muscles of the upper back.

If a bent press is held in the proper position (this position varies in the case of different lifters), the weight will " rise on the latissimus " as I like to phrase it. The triceps muscle should rest crossways upon the latissimus and as the body inclines to the side and front the latissimus muscle hardens and actually elevates the heavy weight. While side pressing is beneficial it does not provide quite as much work for the muscles of the upper sides, but it does cause considerably more leaning to the side and involves the muscles beneficially from a somewhat different angle. The exercise which leads to proficiency in the side or bent press is best known as a shoulder builder but is also wonderful for the upper back. It is a modification of the side press. To practice this movement, take a dumbell and lift it to the shoulder. Stand with the feet about shoulder width apart and step forward approximately six inches with the opposite foot. If you are lifting with the right arm you will stand with that leg straight and the hip thrown to the right for balance; the left knee is somewhat bent and serves chiefly as a balance. As you lean in the direction of the foot on the non-lifting side, push the dumbell to arm's length with the right arm. Straighten your body as your arm is straightened, and then comes perhaps the most important and most beneficial part of the movement for the upper back. Lower the arm slowly so that the bell is kept away from the lifting shoulder. Have the bell turned so that the front end of it is just a bit forward from a line parallel with the shoulders. While lowering the dumbell slowly, deliberately harden the latissimus. The horizontal right arm will gradually lower until it rests upon this muscle. When you learn to perform this movement properly you will find that very little pressing effort is required; you lean forward and the bell goes up almost of its own accord.

While the bent press and the actual side press are lifts in which you should employ heavy weights, the movement I am describing is an exercise and the amount of weight practiced is less important than just how the exercise is done. I have been specializing in the bent press for the last few weeks. I start off each day's training with successive pressing with 50-, 60-, 75- and 100-pound dumbells. I have a 120-pound dumbell and sometimes progress to it but at other times continue to work up using the bar bell. I make my first presses with each weight, not permitting it to touch the body, elevating it with the pressing power and the action of leaning forward. On the second series however I go through the motions in the actual bent press position except that I don't lean far to the side. The arm rests on the latissimus and with a twisting of the dumbell—so that it hangs toward the right eye, as I stated before, with the part of the dumbell toward the head a bit forward of a line parallel with the shoulders—the bells go up with astonishing ease. I pressed a hundred-pound dumbell in that style twenty-two repetitions almost effortlessly until near the end. While all men differ a bit in the position they find best for their individual selves in bent pressing, I have found my best spot to be as I am endeavoring to describe. And this particular method is a splendid developer of the latissimus. I found my coats getting a bit too tight and requiring alterations upon the upper back. You can't do too much lifting, for it will pay great dividends in strength, health and of course the developing of all the muscles.

As the chief function of the latissimus is to draw the arms down and back, as we have already said that swimming, chinning, and rope climbing are good exercises (although not the very best) to develop the muscles of the upper back, notably the latissimus, it is a good plan to rig up an apparatus for the progressive practice of the movements which bring such beneficial effect to the latissimus. You can be sure that if you will faithfully and persistently follow the exercises contained in this and other chapters, you'll be pleased, actually thrilled at the fine results you obtain.

Pulleys should be placed overhead. If you have access to a well-equipped gymnasium such an outfit will probably be present. If not, you can go to the hardware store and obtain two pulleys. Place them overhead, obtain long ropes, handles such as are a part of a cable set or Home Gym and you are ready to proceed. In addition to developing the latissimus, these movements are particularly advantageous in developing the rib-like muscles of the sides, the serratus major and serratus minor. These muscles placed between the ribs really hold them together, so that they are continuous as are the links of a chain. They become very strong and well developed in the powerfully built man, and provide some bulk and increased measurement at the point of the upper chest usually encircled by the tape in taking one's measure.

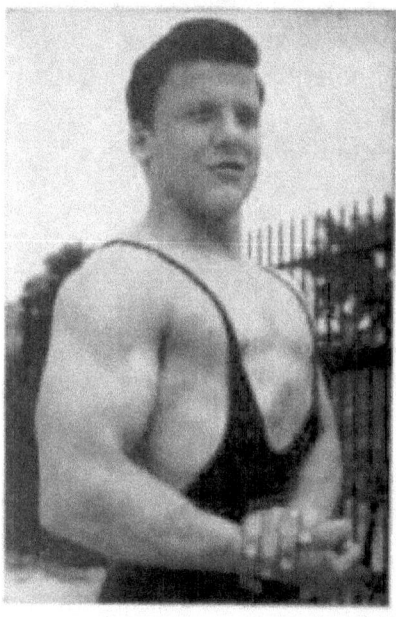

Jack Brace, another young man of the York Bar Bell Club. 17 years of age. Only 5 feet in height, he has built a very strong and attractive physique. Last year he won the Middle Atlantic A. A. U. 123-pound weight lifting title.

The first movement consists of pulling the arms down from overhead sideways, arms straight, exhaling as the arms are lowered, inhaling as they are raised. The inhalation should be performed very deeply and the movements practiced, as is advantageous in nearly all weight exercises, so that you can feel the resistance of the weight every inch of the way. Inhaling slowly and steadily should see the lungs completely inflated when the arms are straight and overhead. Therefore this exercise which is desirable for developing the latissimus also takes rank with the best of the exercises which expand the internal chest or rib box. Not quite the same effect or as good an effect will be had if the weights are pulled, down with the arms extended to the front but it will involve the muscles in a somewhat different angle and of course will be helpful as a developer. This exercise will bring quick results. If you were to measure the width of your back when you first start with this movement you will be surprised to find that you have gained from one to two inches in breadth in a single month's time. And this one to two inches may be the difference between an ordinary appearing physique and one which has the marks of strength and development to an extent which will cause it to attract favorable attention wherever it is seen.

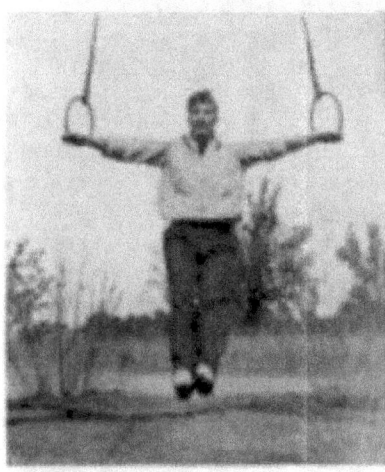

J. E. Kelly, of Kelnoo, S. C. an expert on the Roman rings. This is an exercise which builds a wonderful development of the latissimus.

Another exercise which all of you will not have the desire or the opportunity to practice is one which has helped develop my own latissimus. That is the breaking of chains with the power of the chest. A leather belt is used which comes within six inches of entirely extending around the chest. Two holders of some sort must be fastened to the ends of this belt, then the chain is fastened as tightly as possible between the ends of the belt. Inflate the chest to the limit, the actual breaking of the chain being done with the power of the latissimus muscles. I frequently break four sizes of chains in this manner.

It best attests to the power of the human body, when one considers that soft, moist tissues, the lungs, must be strong enough to force the ribs out sufficiently that when coupled with the strength and power of contraction of the muscles of the chest, a heavy chain is broken. A number of professional strong men break chains, mostly of small size. My chains have been examined by professionals and they agree that the chains have not been tampered with and that they are larger than any chains they have seen broken in a similar manner. I use four sizes of jack chains and at one of our strength exhibitions the heaviest of these chains sustained a weight of 830 pounds. The professional who showed me how to perform this feat of strength told me that he broke two ribs the first time he was trying it. And he was only using a small size chain. Ribs, muscles, and lungs must become strong enough to exert sufficient pressure to break the chain. Many people, realizing that a chain is no stronger than its weakest link, believe that chains have been tampered with before a feat of strength of this sort. I know that mine are new ones right out of the hardware store, and subject them to substantial weight before I attempt to break them—proof that the chain is new, strong and tough.

And before closing this chapter, I cannot overlook the great value of cable expanders, or the Home Gym in developing all of the muscles of the upper body, particularly those of the upper back. Cables have a definite and important place in physical training. Every man interested in physical improvement, the building of strength and a perfect physique, should have a set of cables to use either until he procures a set of weights of his own, or to use in conjunction with a set of weights if he already owns one, or is a member of a club where weights are available.

Invariably when you see a man with a wide-spreading back and mighty shoulders, even if he is a star weight lifter, you will learn upon investigation that he has spent considerable time in cable training. A few years ago Joe Miller, who was definitely one of the strongest men in the world of his weight (only his inability to master best lifting forms prevented him from establishing world's records, although he gathered much fame through being senior national champion of the United States and a member of the Olympic team in 1936) spent a winter in the practice of cable exercises. He had used them in the beginning of his physical training career and they had played an important part in aiding him to set a record in chest growth of twelve full inches in his first year.

Bill Pask.

Bill Lilly.

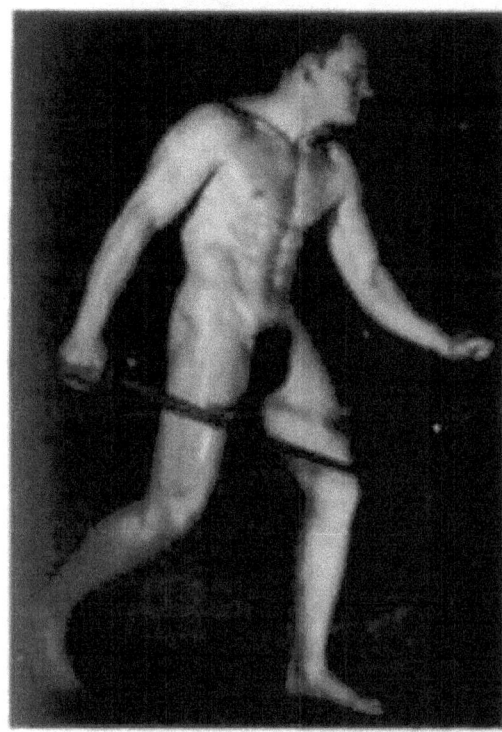

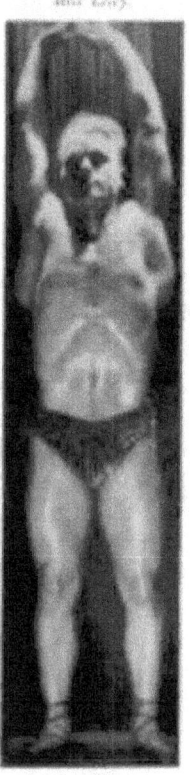

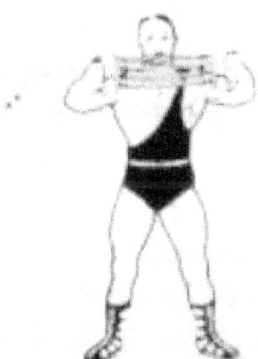

The front pull.

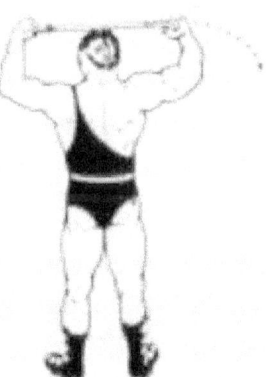

Press behind neck.

He habitually trained in an unheated garage back of his home. Constant training in the cold made his muscles stiff and sore, so he gathered together a real cable outfit and a number of inner tubes which he employed in his training and with which he exercised in his home. He worked hard that winter with chest expanders as they are so often called. In the spring he was stronger than ever as evidenced by his unusual weight lifting ability. Now don't feel that I am trying to tell you that cables will develop the huge muscles of the legs and back to an extent which weights will, but Joe already had a phenomenal lower back and legs, and the cable exercises coupled with his usual work were enough to keep these muscles in shape. He greatly increased the strength of his upper body, notably the muscles of his upper back, which more than offset his lack of weight lifting training. What a back the man had! When the latissimus was tensed his arms stood out to the side at an angle of forty-five degrees. On the Fourth of July he posed in that manner for a newspaper photographer which gave rise to the opinion that weight lifters were so muscle-bound that they couldn't even hang their arms at their sides.

Every cable exercise has a good effect on the muscles of the upper body and there are many of them. But the best of all is an exercise which cannot be practiced with weights. The chest expander is extended at arm's length overhead, then, with arms straight, the cable is stretched so that the arms are pulled down, slightly below shoulder level. You can feel the big muscles of the back in operation as this exercise is practiced. A somewhat similar movement and one that is also highly beneficial for the muscles we are discussing is as follows: Holding the cables overhead with palms out, keep the upper arms level with the shoulders and extended to the sides; the forearms at the start are up in the goose neck position. Straighten the arms. While this movement is admirable for the triceps, you will feel that the latissimus is also heavily involved.

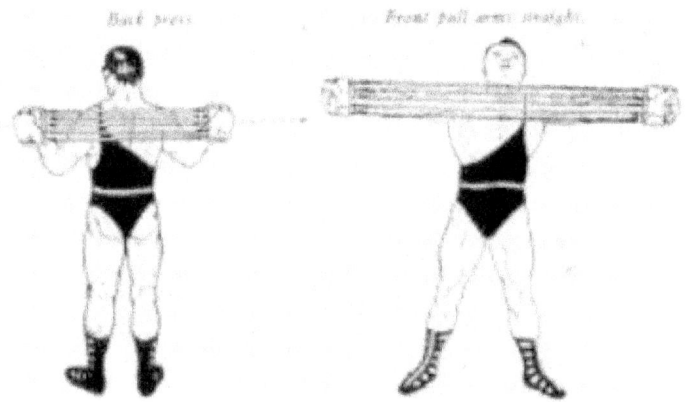

Back press Front pull arms straight

The front press, the archer's movement and the back press are other good cable exercises, particularly the latter, for in this style more resistance can be used than in any other way. Raise the cable up and back so that you have the strands extended across the back, knuckles out, the shoulder blades compressed. Extend the arms steadily to the side, pressing the shoulders out as far as possible. Hardening the muscles as the shoulder blades are brought together will aid in the effects obtained from the movement. Everyone admires a broad, well-muscled back. You'll find that nothing surpasses cable training for broadening the back. Nearly every exercise in which the upper body is involved with cables will develop the muscles of the upper back. The lateral raise with the use of the stirrups has the same effect as a similar movement with weights. Leaning and extending the arms to the side as in the dumbell swing and various forms of rowing motions, all develop the latissimus.

I can't urge you too strongly to include some cable or chest expander exercises in your training. They will fit in between the heavier weight exercises, or on your easy days of training—the days I often term tinkering days, when you perform a multitude of exercises which are not possible to practice on the heavier days of training. You must re-member that to obtain the finest possible development, unusually shapely muscles and greater strength, you cannot perform too many .exercises. Eighteen to twenty-four are not too many on a single day's training. But you should keep a record of the exercises you use in each training period. Don't get in ruts; don't leave out the good ones and don't make a habit of practicing the same movements always. Over a considerable training period be sure that you have included all the exercises which are mentioned in this book as well as others which must be included in a good all-around body conditioning and developing program.

The Muscles of the Chest

THROUGH all of recorded history broad shoulders and a deep, well-muscled chest have been considered to be the mark of physical supremacy. With good shoulders and a well-developed chest, only the addition of a powerful back is needed to possess the appearance of a strong man and to be able to perform the deeds of a strong man.

The world's oldest exercises are dipping movements in various forms, designed primarily to build the muscles of the chest. Many native tribes, particularly the Polynesians, considered to be a type somewhat similar to the Hindus, have splendid development of the pectorals. For so many thousands of years the men of the race from which these men have sprung have had exceptional pectoral development so that it has become an inherited physical characteristic.

What is considered to be the world's oldest exercise is the cat stretch or dipping in various forms. This exercise has been practiced for thousands of years in India. Even today it is one of the chief exercises of the huge and powerful Indian wrestlers. Indian wrestlers, or Hindu wrestlers we might term them, have many generations of wrestlers behind them. Only the best grapplers can continue in the profession and they are duty bound to marry the daughter of another wrestler. With this system of marriage, which corresponds rather closely to specialized breeding of animals, a truly super-race of men has been produced.

In this country we have a long list of men who have been titled world's champion. Jim Londos has held the title for the longest period; Stanislaus Zbyscho has held and lost it the greatest number of times. Strangler Lewis, Dr. Roller, Jenkins, Farmer Burns, Joe Stecher, Earl Caddock, and the more modern wrestlers, Joe Savoldi and Gus Sunnenberg, have held the so-called world's wrestling title. George

Hackenschmidt, now rather an old timer, was champion in 1908 when they still wrestled. Only one of these men journeyed to India to wrestle the champions there—Zbyscho and he was defeated almost faster than one could take a breath.

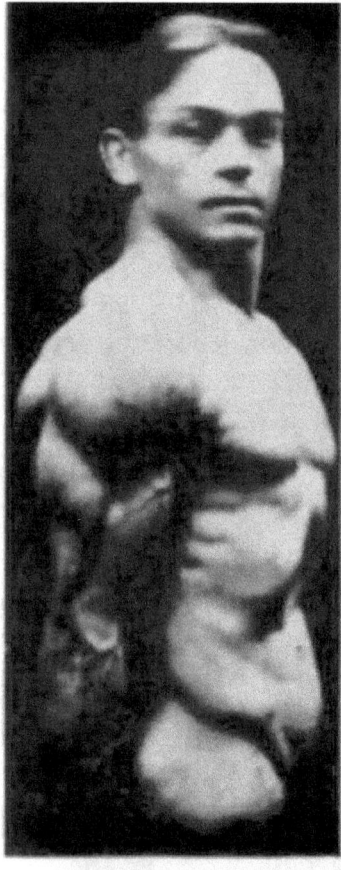
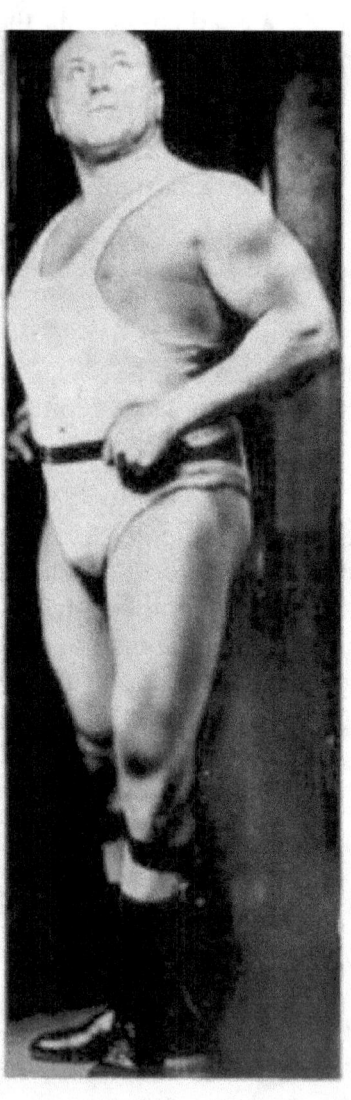

Otto Arco as a young man.

At right, George Hackenschmidt at 60 years of age. He retired from active wrestling and lifting competition in 1908 at the age of 30. He claims not to have exercised since. If his contention that muscles once developed stay with a man throughout his life.

The Hindu wrestlers proved that they excel the world in real wrestling where butting, biting, hitting, kicking, airplane swings and the like are not considered a part of wrestling. These men practice wrestling for hours, and specialize in deep knee bending which, as we will relate anent the rib box expanding exercises, is a real chest developer and the floor dip which is an unusually good pectoral developer. Some time ago two Indian physical culturists established world's records in floor dipping. One of these set a record of 5,130 dips and another exceeded this record by a single dip to make 5,131. The latter man was continually in action for four hours and thirteen minutes, the first performer for four hours and forty-nine minutes. Only many hours, months and years of practice could build such unusual ability in this special exercise.

The constant practice of dipping by the world's oldest races is proof that chest development has long been admired and the possession of big chests has been considered to be the mark of a strong man the world over. While the chest muscles are not the most important muscles of the body from the strength standpoint, they are very important in performing strength feats. They make it possible to hug or crush the body of another, not unlike it is done by Bruin when he becomes real angry. But from the viewpoint of the public, the appearance of these muscles is what counts most. That is why so many physical culturists spend an inordinate amount of time in pectoral exercises. They know that a well-developed pair of these muscles will be so unusual that it will excite favorable attention everywhere. Not only when in bathing or athletic costume but in any form of clothing, the high, round, full chest will be particularly impressive.

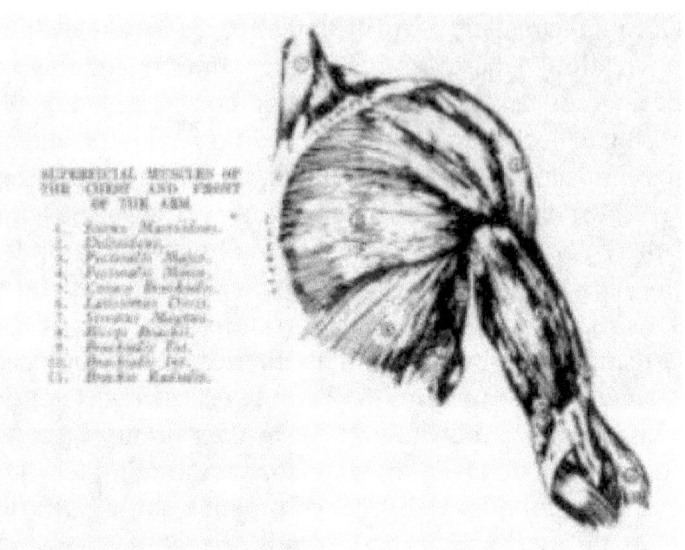

Some of the greats of the past attained their chief fame through the well-rounded, highly developed chest muscles they displayed in all their photos. Antone Matysek, Tony Sansone, Tony Massimo, A. Passanent, and Earl Liederman displayed unusual pectoral development. Many of the more famous Liederman pupils followed their leader and built for themselves chest muscles which added to their fame and gave them universal recognition as strong and perfectly built men. Before going on with the means to develop the pectoral muscles it will be well to consider them anatomically first.

First is the pectoralis major, which arises from the anterior surface of the sternal half of the .clavicle, the anterior surface of the sternum, the cartilages of the true ribs and the aponeurosis of the external oblique. The broad flat fibres which cover the entire upper chest area converge and form a thick mass which is inserted by a flat tendon into the crest of the greater tubercle of the humerus.

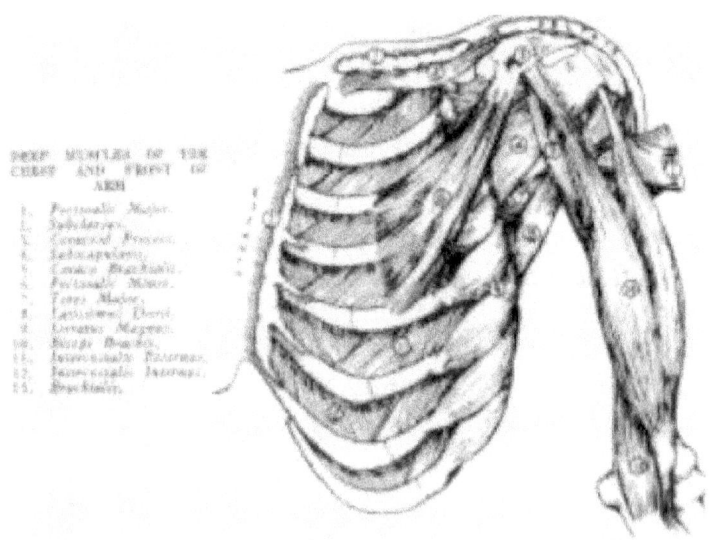

When the arm has been raised, the pectorals, acting with the latissimus dorsi muscles and the teres major, draw the arms down to the side of the chest. Acting alone they adduct and draw the arm across the chest and rotate it inward. From this brief description you can see why the two hands pull over while lying, and the lateral raise lying, ending by folding the arms over the chest, are prime exercises for developing these muscles.

The pectoralis minor lies underneath and is entirely covered by the pectoralis major. It arises from the outer margins and the outer surfaces of the third, fourth and fifth ribs near their cartilages, and is inserted into the caracoid process of the scapula. Its work is to depress the point of the shoulder and rotate the scapula downward. In forced inspiration the pectoral muscles aid in drawing the ribs upward and expanding the chest.

The serratus magnus arises from the outer surface and superior borders of the upper eight or nine ribs and the intercostals between them. The fibres pass upward and backward and are inserted in various portions of the ventral surface of the scapula. It carries the scapula forward and raises the vertical Border of the bone as in pushing. It assists the trapezius in raising the acromium process and supporting weights on the shoulder. It also assists the deltoid in raising the arm.

The intercostals are found filling the spaces between the ribs. Each muscle consists of two layers, one external and one internal, and as there are eleven intercostal spaces on each side, and two muscles in each space, therefore there are forty-four intercostal muscles. The fibres of these muscles run in opposite directions.

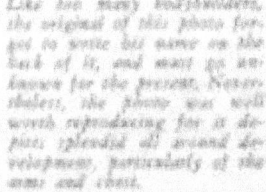

Like too many bodybuilders, the original of this photo forgot to write his name on the back of it, and must go unknown for the present. Nevertheless, the photo was well worth reproducing for it depicts splendid all around development, particularly of the arms and chest.

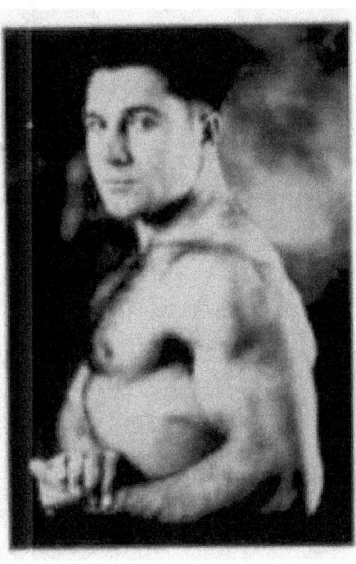

The external intercostals extend from the tubercles of the ribs behind to the cartilages of the ribs in front, where they end in membranes which connect with the sternum. Each arises from the lower border of a rib and is inserted into the upper border of the fifth rib. The direction of the fibres is obliquely downward. The internal intercostals extend from the sternum to the angle of the ribs and are connected to the vertebral column. Each arises from the inner surface of a rib and is inserted into the upper portion of the rib below.

The direction of the fibres is obliquely downward and opposite to the direction of the external intercostals.

There is some disagreement among experts as to the operation of the intercostal muscles. One expert states that the internal and external intercostals contract simultaneously and prevent the intercostal spaces from being pushed outward or drawn inward during respiration. Another classes them as inspiratory.

There are twelve little-known muscles known as the levatores costarum which arise from the tranverse processes of the vertebrae. They pass obliquely downward and lateralward like the external intercostals. Each one is inserted into the outer surface of the rib, just below the vertebra from which it takes its origin. It is believed that these muscles act as rotators and lateral flexors of the vertebral column.

Of the muscles we have briefly described the pectoral muscles are of chief interest to most body builders. In fact many of them don't know that they even have the other muscles, don't know the serratus magnus or the intercostals from the Aurora Borealis. But those familiar with body building and the well-developed masculine physique know and admire these little-known muscles. Any advanced muscle control artist can exhibit these muscles. In themselves they are not so important from the strength angle and they don't add much to the appearance of the physique. The thin fellow has only ribs to show and can't find them. The man who is even slightly well upholstered won't see them, but when you can detect these muscles plainly in a well-developed state, you will know that you are looking at a real man, a man who is strong inside and out, who possesses great virility and internal power, splendid digestion, good elimination, endurance and all desirable physical qualities. Not that these muscles control the functions I have just mentioned, but the man who has well-developed serratus magnus and intercostals is carrying the proof that he has performed the sort of exercises which build internal strength. While he has been developing these little-known external muscles, he has brought to a high stage of perfection the better-known external muscles and has been building the power of the internal organs.

Any man who has transformed his body from the too thin, too weak, too fat class, through weight training, knows what the acquisition of these muscles has meant to him. He knows that he feels better, that he has more pep, greater endurance, that he is starved before meals and can eat like a bear, he knows that he is never constipated, that he doesn't have headaches or even colds, that he is never ill, that he is light on his feet, cheerful and happy. You can be sure that any man who has well-developed serratus magnus, intercostals and external obliques, which are far enough down the sides to be included in the discussion of the midsection, has done a great deal of vigorous bending, twisting, and endurance work. He has built his internal powers and improved the action of all the organs and glands. A good all-around body-building program, including heavy work and weight lifting with specializing upon the muscles this volume deals with, will bring these little-known muscles of the chest to a point where they are plainly noticeable.

As the pectorals are really a three-part muscle which spreads out fanwise from the arm and shoulder, a diversity of exercises is required to develop them fully. Designed to draw the arm downward and forward, exercises which develop the latissimus are also important in their development.

Back to our discussion of dipping. This is one of the best exercises to develop the pectorals. Plain floor dipping, unless you progress to one arm dipping, is not intensive enough to bring the pectorals to the peak of development. When carried on into the hundreds and thousands of repetitions as some Hindu specialists have done, it is not unlike the continued action of a marathon race. It will cause the muscles to be hard, thin and stringy, rather than full and rounded as desired.

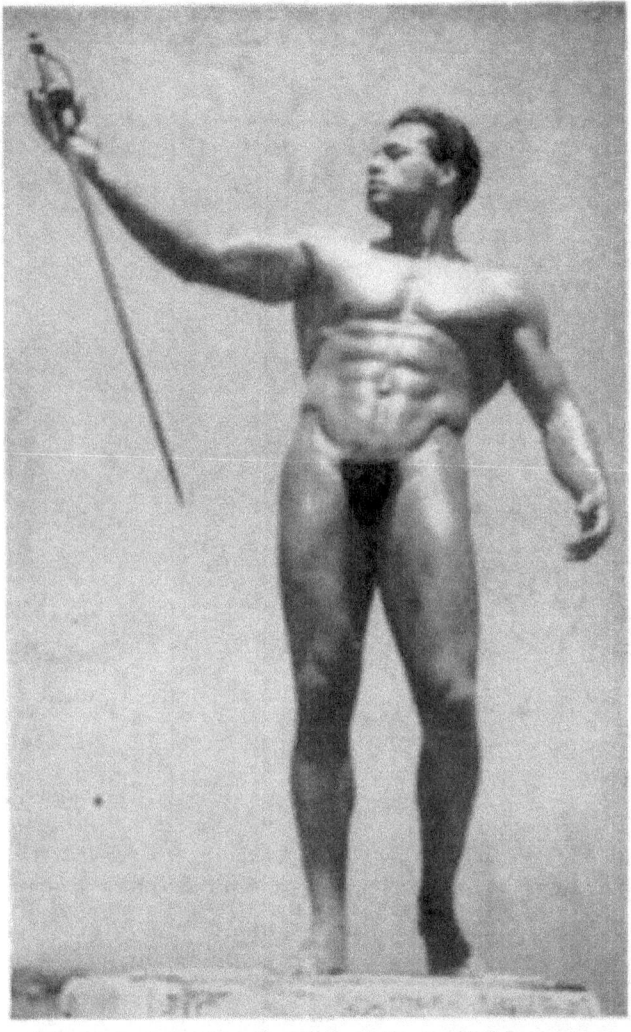

Chick Deutch, of Brooklyn, N. Y. Invariably one of the place winners in best built man contests. He's believed to have the best developed abdominals in the nation, and it can be plainly seen that he excels in chest development as well.

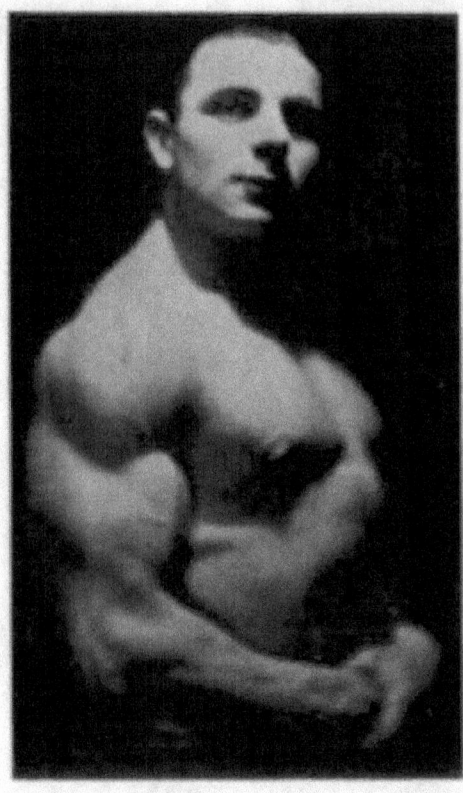

The exercise of dipping can be greatly improved by dipping with the aid of three chairs or three boxes, a hand on each chair, the feet on another. It is advisable to have the feet raised higher than the hands if this is convenient. Dipping between chairs gives you a great range of movement. With the feet raised, more resistance is supplied to the arms and of course the pectorals. This movement can be made progressive by tying weights to the waist. It was considered of sufficient value that quite recently it was offered as the " Exercise of the Month " in Strength and Health magazine. Some men make the movement even more vigorous by having a child or a light training mate sit upon the shoulders. It is a real exercise when performed against such resistance.

Men who are skilled hand balancers practice this movement balanced upon two boxes with the body in the hand balance position. Or if not so adept at balancing, dip from the hand stand position with the feet against the wall. Dipping upon parallel bars is another means to develop these muscles. Here we have three distinctly different positions of dipping: feet raised overhead, feet hanging and feet at shoulder level. These three positions will develop the pectorals in an outstanding manner. Tony Sansone has done a lot of parallel bar dipping, and Elmer Farnham who is noted for his pectoral development has specialized in all forms of dipping. He does not specialize at the present time, but his exceptionally well developed pectorals bear the mark of ample dipping at the inception of his physical training career.

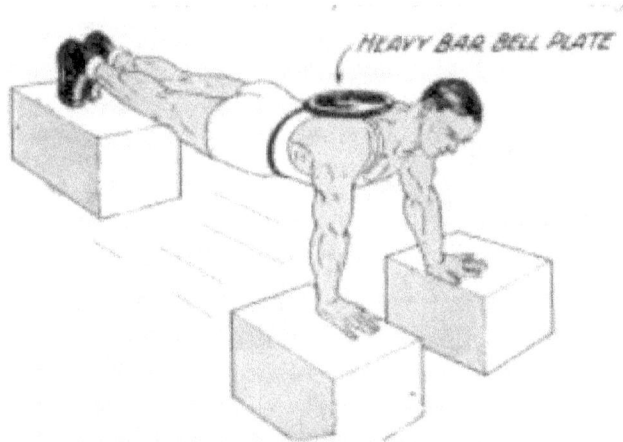

Elmer excels at another form of dipping. Lying flat upon his face, with arms extended to the front, arms straight, he raises his body approximately a foot from the floor. He has done this with ninety-two pounds, and certainly it has promoted the strength and development of his pectorals.

The overhead pulleys that you have rigged up for the development of the latissimus will serve well in pectoral development. There is this difference however: Your back should be to the wall in pectoral exercises, and face to the wall in latissimus movements. Be very careful to hold the arms straight and perform the movements correctly so that the muscles involved will receive the maximum of benefit. Pulley weights, so often called chest weights, are of advantage in developing the chest muscles. They are to be found in most gymnasiums. You can construct your own if you desire, or you can be satisfied with the results which are obtained through bar bell, dumbell and cable training, which I can assure you will be worthy, if you persist in your efforts.

The best known and the best chest-developing exercise of them all is the two arm pull over. This can be practiced while lying upon the floor or on a bench or two boxes. Greater range of movement can be had in this latter movement, and greater range of movement has a better effect from the development standpoint. As a breathing exercise only a moderate weight should be employed as we will explain more fully in the chapter devoted to expanding the chest.

As a muscle builder, employ the weight you can properly handle. While in the muscle-building exercise, only a quarter circle is made with the arms and the bar. From far back of head to thighs is best in this breathing exercise. Use a heavier weight in this movement and develop your muscles to the fullest extent. Keeping the arms entirely straight, continue the movement steadily; try to keep your back flat against the floor or the bench or boxes. A man who can pull over one hundred pounds is really strong and will have pectoral development to prove it.

The next best movement is somewhat similar but performed this time with two dumbells. It is known as the lateral raise lying. Raise the dumbells to arm's length above the chest, knuckles out. Lower the bells, keeping arms straight throughout until they are a bit lower than level with

174

shoulders. This movement can be varied a bit by crossing the arms after they have reached a point above the body.

In this movement you are limited by the strength of the muscles on the inside of the elbows and the shoulders. So an even better chest developing exercise is a form of flying movement. If you have partaken of a dinner of squab, pheasant, quail, duck or other wild bird, you must have been impressed with the tremendous size and depth of the chest or breast muscles in relation to the size of the bird. Flying as they do for long distances, frequently at great speed, they have developed breast muscles which make up a large part of the muscular bulk of their small bodies. It is evident that some form of flying exercise will advantageously benefit the human body builder.

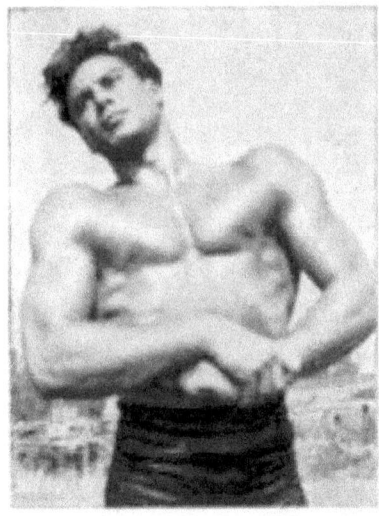

Bill Fisher, of Philadelphia, showing the results of two years of York Bar Bell training and cable exercising. He has a 48-inch expanded chest, performs a shoulder bridge press with 350 pounds and a wrestler's bridge press with 250. By profession he is a commercial artist.

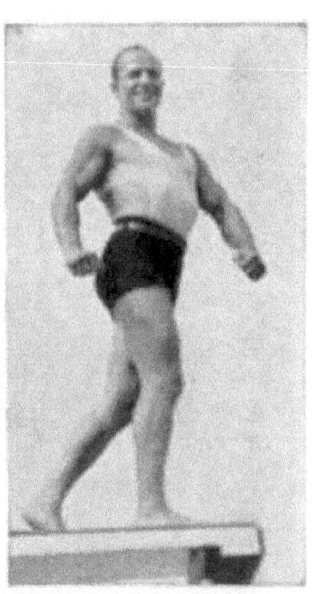

Jack Russell, long famed as the possessor of one of America's best physiques. He has written many articles on physical training which have appeared in international publications.

Two or three times as much weight can be used in this flying exercise as in the lateral raise lying. The elbows are kept bent and a movement employed similar to flying, with the dumbells touching above at the center of the body and ranging out as far as they can extend from the sides with bent arms. The range of movement can be varied by moving the dumbells from a position at the side of the shoulders along the entire range of the body until opposite the abdomen. Jake Hitchin, who was one of the originators of this movement, has used ioo pounds in each hand and has been rewarded by huge, shapely, powerful breast muscles.

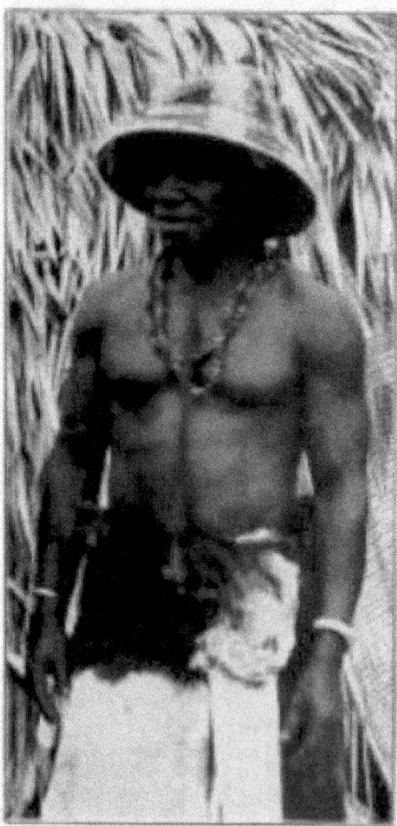

All natives, whether red, black or brown, whether African, Polynesian or Oriental, are the possessors of very well developed chest muscles. It is natural for the pectoral or breast muscles to be well developed. Only lack of use for generation after generation has caused the white man's pectorals to deteriorate.

Another of my favorites (you'll soon think that all are my favorites) is the two hands press with bar bell or dumbells while lying upon boxes or bench. While I enjoy many exercises, the upright rowing motion with dumbells and the press on box or bench take rank well at the head of the list with me. By alternately pressing two dumbells or pressing them simultaneously a somewhat different action is given to the pectoral muscles than in dipping. It is a splendid breathing exercise too as you'll read later. But with the bar bell you can really handle a substantial poundage and obtain favorable results commensurate with the effort expended. Recently I performed ten movements in this style with 200 pounds. Poor leverage in the military or continental style of pressing does not seem to hinder me when pressing in this position. Some years ago most of us were much surprised to learn that I could outpress all but three or four of our champions in this position, men who could actually outpress me a hundred pounds in the military position—my 190 as compared to 300 or more of men such as Davis, Grimek and Stanko.

While lying upon boxes there are many variations of the lateral laise and the two arm pull over which serve well with dumbells. Alternate forward and lateral raise, holding the weights at arm's length above the head and then dropping both of them first to right, then back to center, then to left. Or a twisting and turning movement such as the following: Thrust the dumbells to straight arms back of head. Holding palms up and keeping arms straight bring them down past the waist and to the thighs, permitting the arms to turn so that the knuckles are now up; cross them, bringing them forward, close to the body and back of the head to the original position. Continue this movement until tired.

Two favorably known appliances lend themselves well to chest muscle building. The first of these is the Giant

Crusher Grip. It brings into action the crushing muscles of the body and as this is one of the prime purposes of the pectoral muscles and as they can't be reached in quite the same way with any other equipment, a giant crusher grip should be included in the training equipment of every ambitious physical culturist. At one time I took a mail order course of exercises offered by one of the champion wrestlers of the day. The training equipment which came with this course was a form of crusher grip. How I enjoyed using this piece of equipment and I feel that I was permanently rewarded by chest increases both in size and development. There is a fair range of movement with the Giant Crusher Grip.

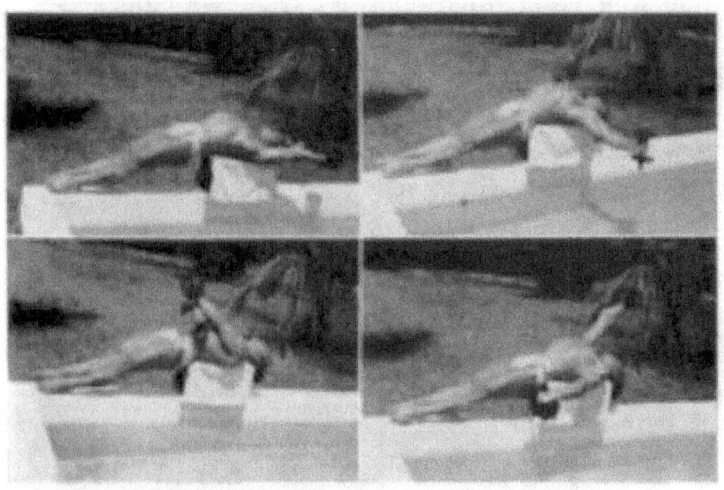

Some of the best chest development exercises. Anyone who has seen John Grimek training will note that he spends a good share of his training time at the practice of the exercises shown here. They have contributed a large share of his exceptional rib box and pectoral development.

The Iron Shoe, while working in exactly the opposite manner, nevertheless exerts considerable action with resulting benefit to the chest muscles.

As cables were commonly called chest expanders, and as the best cable pullers all have good pectorals it is evident that they are highly beneficial in building this important

178

part of the anatomy. Most of the exercises offered in the chapter on building the latissimus provide almost equal benefit to the pectorals. If you do not have weights, are so situated that it is objectionable to use them, usually in hotels, boarding houses or apartments where the least noise is objectionable, you can practice all forms of lateral raises and two arm pull overs with the Home Gym cable set and attachments.

As a general thing, although I say that any exercise is better than no exercise, I do not favor resistance exercises — where one arm works against another. Through untold generations of human beings, definite, coordinated muscle movements have been followed. The brain has learned to direct these movements in a normal manner. But work one set of muscles against another, such as in curling with one arm as the other resists in a pressing action, and the best results are not obtained. Countless men have reported headaches and dizziness from these movements without knowing why. The fact that it is contrary to the laws of normal movement which our own ancestors' bodies had become accustomed to, long before the dawn of recorded history, accounts for this confusion when the mind is unable to properly work in conjunction with this new type of movement and the mental bewilderment causes dizziness and even headaches.

But I have several pectoral-developing exercises to offer which are not detrimental to one's feelings. Extend the arms in front of the body, palms together. Maintaining a vigorous pressure with the palms, raise the arms to full length overhead, keeping the arms straight throughout. Momentarily relax, then continue down with the arms until a position at the thighs is reached. Continue this movement until tired.

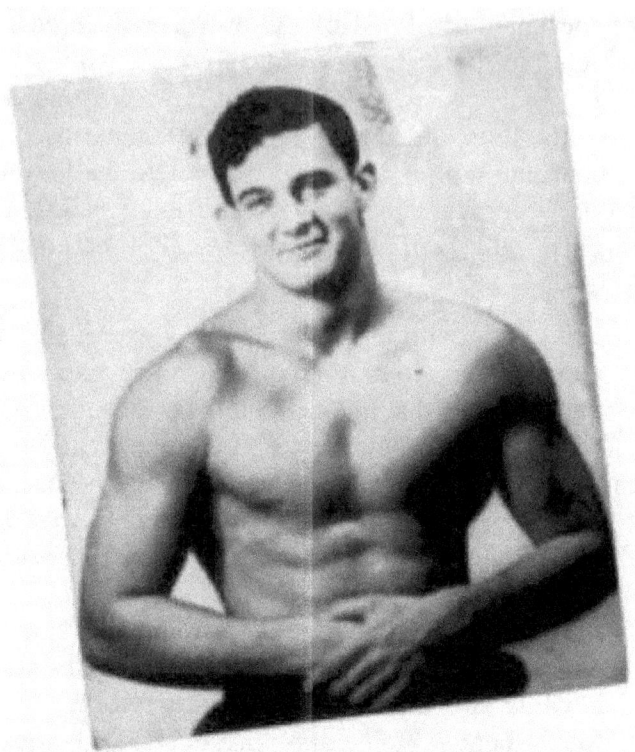

Jack Reid, of Miami Beach, Florida, was a victim of infantile paralysis. He spent long years with his legs in braces. His weight was only 120 pounds when he seriously started at progressive training. Most of the muscles he removed, developing himself to the splendid physique shown here and a body weight of 185 pounds, resulted from the use of cables. When such effects have been obtained by the legions of men who started with physical handicaps, it certainly should make any normal men who do not build their bodies ashamed of themselves. Don't you think?

Another similar movement is to place the hands with palms together, fingers extended right in front of the chest. The elbows are bent. Keeping close to the body, and pressing hard with the hands and arms, raise the hands to arm's length over the head, relax momentarily and come down to a position below the chest. And a third: The starting position is the same as that in exercise No. 2. The right hand presses hard, the left resists but not quite as strongly as the right presses and the left hand is pushed far to the left. Then the left pushes hard to the right and the movement is continued. Maintain a heavy and steady pressure of the hands. This will tighten the pectorals and will cause them to grow in size and strength.

The famous old time strong men and many men of the present control their chest muscles frequently, causing them to move together or alternately. To learn this movement the exercise I have just offered is best. But tighten and relax the chest muscles more frequently and soon you will attain such control over them that you can move them at will in any position.

Persistence in practicing these recommended exercises and others which may suggest themselves to you will add an inch or two to the depth of your chest muscles and, in line with the former reasoning offered once before that the circumference of a circle is three and one-seventh times the diameter, an increase in diameter of one or two inches will mean an increased chest girth of three to six inches.

It is evident from these several chapters concerning the development of the muscles of the chest that practice of the exercises offered will give you a chest that stretches the tape to many more inches, but the real way to a bigger chest is to build the rib box, deepen it from front to rear in particular, and that phase of physical improvement will be our discussion in the next chapter.

Expanding the Rib Box

WHILE this book has already contained much of importance, development of the rib box ranks ahead of muscle building. As has been our habit up to this point we will include an anatomical discussion of the nomenclature of the rib box before going on with exercises to develop the bony framework of the chest.

The part of the body which we familiarly know as the rib box is really named the thorax. It is a bony cage formed by the sternum and the costal cartilages in front, the ribs on each side, and the bodies of the thoracic vertebrae behind. It is roughly cone-shaped, being narrow above and broad from below, flattened somewhat in the front and shorter in front than in the back. In infancy the chest is more rounded or barrel-like, the width from shoulder to shoulder and the depth from sternum to vertebra being about equal. The width increases out of proportion to depth as growth progresses. The thorax supports the bones of the shoulder girdle and upper extremities and contains and protects the heart and lungs, the organs of respiration and circulation.

The sternum or breastbone is a flat, narrow bone about six inches long, situated in the median line in the front of the chest. It develops as three separate parts. The upper part is named the manubrium; the middle and largest part is named the gladiolus; the lowest portion is termed the ensiform or xiphoid process. On both sides of the manubrium and body are notches for the reception of the sternal ends of the upper seven costal cartilages. The xiphoid process has no ribs attached to it, but affords attachment to some of the abdominal muscles.

The sternum consists of several unossified portions at birth, the body alone developing from four centers. Union in the centers of the body begins at about puberty and proceeds from below upward until at about twenty-five years of age they are united. The xiphoid process sometimes becomes joined to the body by thirty years of age, more often after forty. In more advanced life the manubrium may become joined to the body by bony tissue. Posture and dietary hygiene have much to do with shaping the sternum and the thoracic cavity.

Situated on each side of the thoracic cavity are the ribs, twenty-four in number. They are elastic arches of bone consisting of a body or shaft and two extremities, the posterior or vertebral, and the anterior or sternal. Each rib is connected with the thoracic vertebra by the head and tubercle of the posterior extremity. The head fits into a facet formed on the body of one vertebra, or formed by the adjacent bodies of two vertebrae; the tubercle articulates with the transverse processes. Strong ligaments surround and bind these articulations but permit slight gliding movements between them.

The anterior extremities of each of the first seven pairs are connected with the sternum in front by means of the costal cartilages. They are called true ribs. The remaining five pairs are termed false ribs. Of these the upper three, eighth, ninth and tenth, are attached in front to the costal cartilages of the next rib above. The two lowest are unattached in front, and are termed floating ribs. The convexity of the rib is turned outward so as to give roundness to the sides of the chest and increase the size and capacity. Each rib slopes downward from its posterior attachment, so that its sternal end is considerably lower than its vertebral. The lower border of each rib is grooved for the accommodation of the intercostal nerves and blood vessels. The spaces left between the ribs are termed the intercostal spaces.

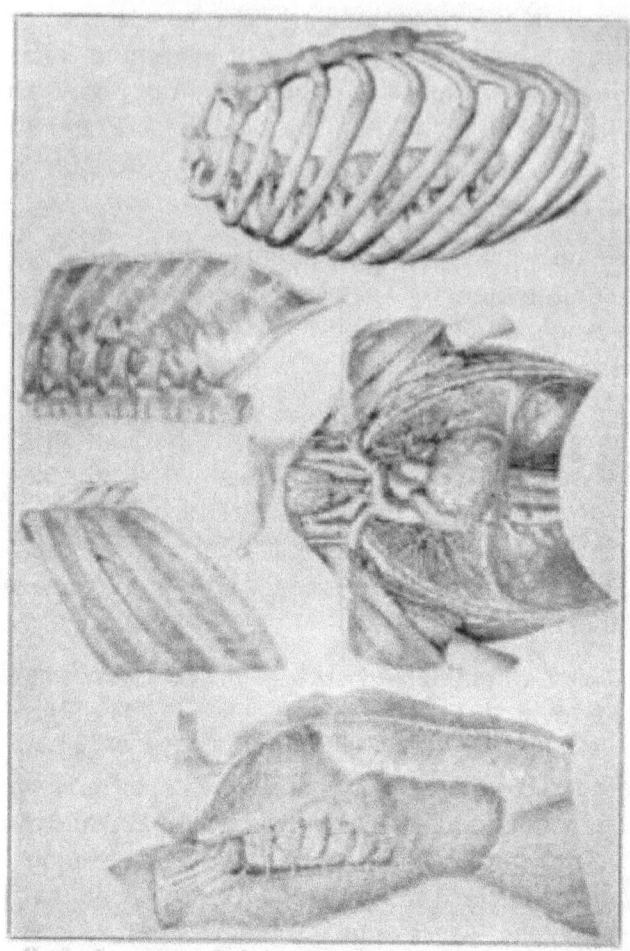

Included as a part of the chest are the bones of the shoulder girdle, the clavicle or collarbone, the scapula or shoulder bone. There are two of each. The clavicles articulate with the sternum in front but in the rear the scapulae are connected to the trunk by muscles only. The shoulder girdle stretches to attach the bones of the upper extremity to the axial skeleton.

The collarbone has a double curvature and is placed horizontally at the upper and anterior part of the thorax, just above the first rib. It articulates with the sternum by its inner extremity, which is called the sternal extremity. In the female, the clavicle is generally less curved, smoother, shorter, and more, slender than in the male. In those persons who perform considerable manual labor which brings the muscles connected with this bone into constant use, it acquires considerable bulk.

The shoulder blade is a large, flat bone, triangular in shape, placed between the second and seventh ribs on the back part of the thorax. It is unevenly divided on its dorsal surface by a very prominent ridge, the spine of the scapulae, which terminates in a large triangular projection called the acromium process. At the head of the shoulder blade is a shallow socket, the glenoid cavity, which receives the head of the humerus.

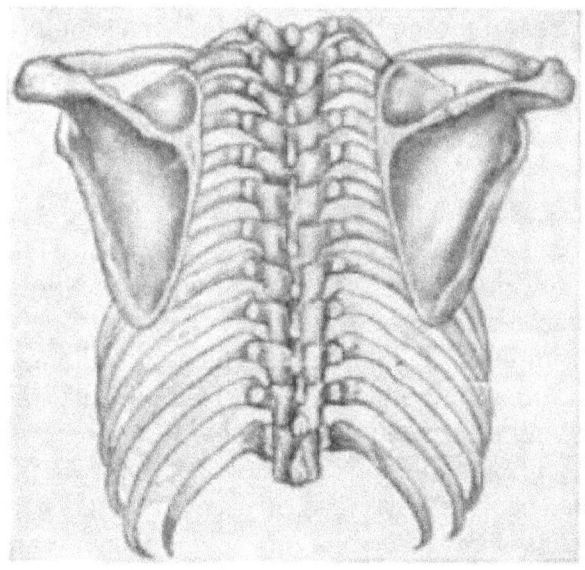

Posterior view of the rib box which illustrates the position of the scapula and shoulder girdle

As the arms are employed in all chest-developing exercises we will include the humerus or upper arm bone in our discussion. The humerus is the longest and largest bone of the upper limb. The upper extremity consists of a rounded head joined to the shaft by a constricted neck and of two eminences called the greater and lesser tubercles, between which is the intertubercular groove. The constricted neck above the tubercles is called the anatomical neck, and that below the tubercles the surgical neck, because it is so often fractured. The head articulates with the glenoid cavity of the shoulder blade. The lower extremity of the bone is flattened from before backward and ends below in an articular surface which is divided by a ridge into a lateral eminence called the capitulum and a medial portion called the trochlea. The capitulum is rounded and articulates with the depression on the head of the radius. The trochlea articulates with the ulna.

From this brief description it is evident that the entire construction of the rib box, collarbones and shoulder blades is sufficiently flexible to permit of considerable adjustment and enlargement in size. Some of the parts do not become ossified or permanently hardened and attached until well past the age of forty. We can easily understand how muscles, tendons and ligaments which attach these bones to one another can permit of considerable adjustment when books of anatomy inform us that in those persons who perform considerable manual labor, which brings the muscles connected with the bone into constant action, the bone—in this case the collarbone—acquires considerable bulk. When the bones in individuals past maturity can enlarge as so often is shown by growth in wrist and ankles, definite proof that the bone has become larger, it is easy to understand how adjustments can take place which greatly wider, the shoulders, deepen and enlarge the chest. It has always been my contention that a man can continue to improve until he is at least fifty years of age, that he can stay near his peak for many more years after he has reached that age. The nose and ears of humans grow until the age of one hundred if that advanced age is attained—proving that the body is still capable of growth when an advanced age is reached.

Thousands of cases of enlarged chests and broadened shoulders have resulted from progressive training when an age of maturity has arrived. In the 1940 Strength and Health Self-Improvement Contest, with six thousand men taking part (at least this many men formally entered the contest; there may have been a great many others), a great many cases were brought to my attention of men who were past the age of forty who gained three or four inches in chest girth during this period. Part of this gain would have been muscular improvement but a goodly share of it was an adjustment in the rib box and the shoulders.

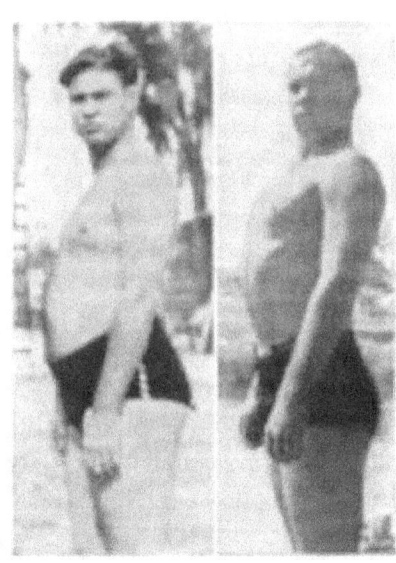

Paul Cressman of Selinsgrove, who made an improvement in his build during the three months of the great Strength and Health Self-Improvement Contest. He reduced his weight 34 pounds, yet increased the circumference of his chest by a full five inches. Starting with a waist of 38 and a chest of 40 inches he ended the contest with 43-inch chest and 33-inch waist.

My own gain of fourteen inches since I reached the age of twenty-one—from thirty-six to fifty—probably would have been even more rapid if I had been so situated that I could train regularly. The first five of these years went by with only the practice of athletics. When I learned of bar bells

187

back in 1923 I was so situated that I traveled constantly and could not train as regularly as I liked. My gains were slow, but sure. Consider the case of a famous physical trainer and author—Reverend H. B. Lange, at one time director of physical education at Notre Dame University, who took up bar bell training at the age of thirty, at which time he had a thirty-six-inch chest. He progressed, in the next few years, to more than a fifty-inch chest. I recently had the opportunity to talk to some enthusiasts from Notre Dame and they said that the reverend professor, now well advanced in years, is still a splendid physical specimen.

At least we can all be encouraged, regardless of pre^nt strength and development, by what so many men in the past have accomplished. With similar exercises and similar effort there is no reason why any man cannot greatly improve in chest girth, chest strength and health.

Writers of the past have been divided as to what is the best exercise to enlarge the rib box, whether the two hands pull over practiced as a breathing exercise or the deep knee bend with enforced breathing is the best exercise. It has always been my contention that both are essential. The deep knee bend first causes a condition of breathlessness; then when followed by some form of two hands pull over, while there is a great need for air to bring the bodily processes back to normal after the great exertion they have undergone, the two hands pull over does its work well. Without the deep knee bend, while the pull over will be beneficial, I believe that it does not serve as fully as when following vigorous exercise which leaves one breathless.

In all the York courses—the four bar bell courses, the four dumbell courses, the cable courses—some form of pull over follows the deep knee bend. The courses all start off with an easy warming up exercise, to speed up the action of heart and lungs. Then two movements, some form of curl and press, which are not too difficult, then the hardest exercise of them all while the body builder is fresh—the deep knee bend—and then some form of pull over, or lateral raise while lying upon bench or box; at least a good breathing exercise.

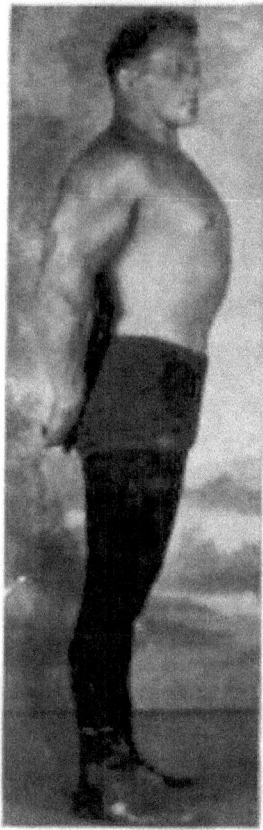

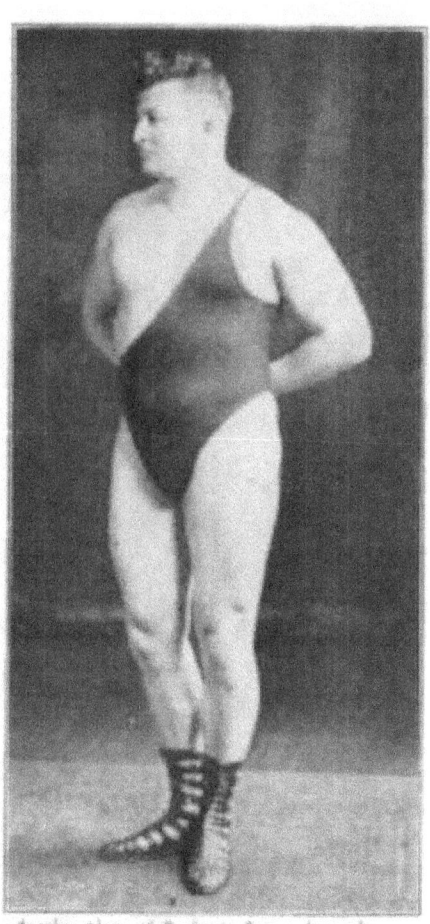

Below: Henry Steinborn, the "Strongest man in wrestling," as a young man. Once weighs recently at the age of 47 we saw him wrestle a thrilling match with Londos. He clean and jerked 375 pounds for a new world's record when this photo was taken.

Another photo of Professor Large, formerly of Notre Dame, the man who took up foot ball training at thirty, and built his chest from 36 inches to 50. He possesses a symmetrical physique as it is evident that he made gains all over.

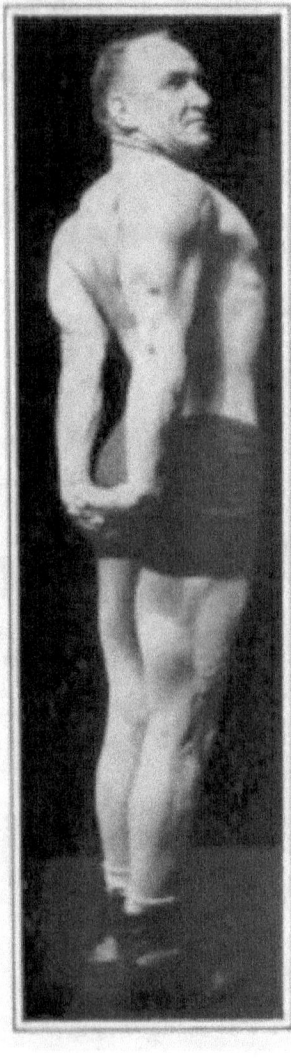

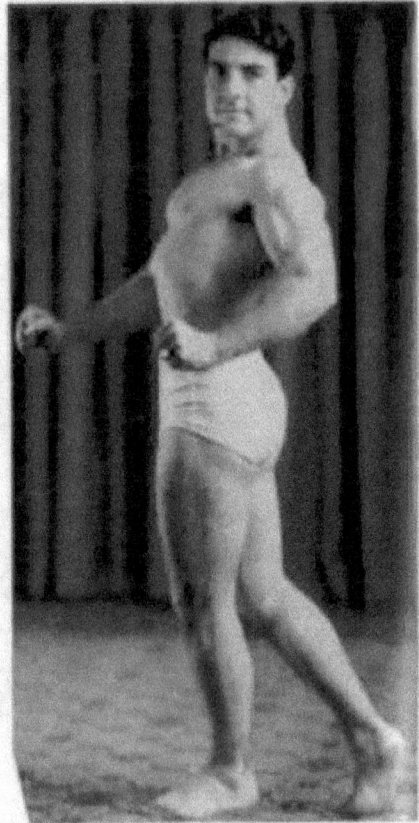

Walter Donald, who first came to the attention of the physical training public by posing for all the exercise photos in a famous old book called "Super Strength."

Recent photo of Tony Terlazzo, world's champion weight lifter. Tony is an office executive, 29 years of age and married.

There are a variety of ways to perform the deep knee bend: as a muscle builder, as an endurance builder and as a chest builder. It is at times necessary to handle very heavy poundages to strengthen the muscles, tendons and ligaments to their limit. This very heavy weight will not permit many consecutive movements. One of the original York principles—the Heavy and Light system—comes into play here. The exercise is performed with all the weight you can handle seven, or eight times. After a short breathing spell, ten to twenty per cent of the weight is removed and seven or eight additional deep knee bends are practiced. Sometimes three times five, five bends, a rest, five more, another rest and then another five more is practiced. This form of deep knee bending will build great strength in the muscles and attachments involved, but it is not as good a muscle builder or chest developer as other methods I will describe.

In building muscle a certain number of repetitions is required to make sufficient demands upon the muscle involved that an increased quantity of blood rushes to the rescue of the working muscle. The blood responds quickly and it has always been my belief that ten or preferably twelve movements are needed to attract the blood which will replenish the energy put forth in the particular muscle group which is being used in the exercise. For muscle and strength building I recommend ten or twelve movements, fifteen at the most. It is my belief that, if more than fifteen movements are practiced in a muscle-building exercise, only endurance and muscles of moderate size will result. The muscles will become just strong enough to overcome the work they are asked to do and a bit more as a reserve. Therefore I prefer to have my pupils use more weight and fewer movements, providing they are between ten and fifteen, on the normal training day; a different system as I outlined in developing strength in muscles and ligaments.

I make this explanation so that there will not be confusion in the system of chest building I am offering in this chapter. Substantially as I have outlined above, the various recommendations I have made are offered in the York courses, Heavy and Light—ten to fifteen for muscle building, and more for easier movements such as shoulder shrug, raise on toes, straddle hop or various forms of breathing exercises. Twenty has been the recommended number of movements for the various forms of breathing exercises.

You may, if you are an advanced bar bell man, be capable of a single bend with three hundred and fifty pounds. Possibly you can use three hundred in the heavy and light method of training, and two hundred and fifty for fifteen repetitions. In this method of using the deep knee bend to create the demands which will result in greater need for oxygen with resulting gains in chest measurement, a weight of not more than body weight will be sufficient—certainly not over a few pounds more than body weight, for the benefit of the exercise will be obtained from the manner in which the movement is performed, rather than the weight employed. But you must have sufficient weight to make demands and induce breathlessness which is an essential part of employing the deep knee bend as a breathing exercise.

With the normal style of deep knee bending, only one deep breath is taken between each bend, unless toward the end you have become so breathless that yoil pause for two or three breaths until you complete the planned number of repetitions. But in employing the deep knee bend as a breathing exercise you will use this system from the beginning, even before you become breathless.

You'll find it necessary to get in the habit of breathing through the mouth if you don't already use that style, for you will be inhaling and exhaling a greater quantity of air than can properly go through your nostrils in a reasonable time, when the effort becomes great. So start right out with a weight not much more, if any more, than your body weight; we'll say two hundred pounds even for the star deep knee bender who has a record of three hundred and fifty. Take a deep breath; exhale completely; take another deep breath; exhale completely; take another deep breath, trying to compress all the air possible in the lungs and to widen the rib box as much as possible, then squat on full lungs, exhaling as you rise.

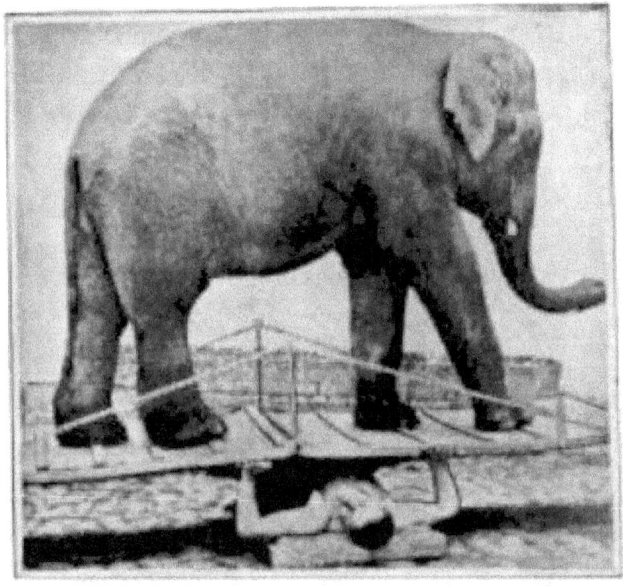

By supporting this 4,000-pound elephant the powerful man underneath illustrates just how phenomenally strong this flexible but uniquely constructed rib box or thorax is.

Take three deep breaths as described previously, then another deep knee bend on full lungs. Continue this for a full twenty counts. If you are new to such a program, during the program or at least within a day or two, your chest will ache slightly. Don't let this disturb you, for adjustments will be taking place in your lungs and rib box; you will actually be experiencing a condition which you could term growing pains. The chest should respond to this specialization in chest exercises so that you should gain in chest measurement from one to four inches in a single month even if you are an experienced bar bell man who has long been practicing the deep knee bend and the two arm pull over. You are practicing these movements in a somewhat different manner now, breathing hundreds of times to the fullest extent in each training period and naturally you'll feel it.

Unaccustomed muscles become a bit stiff through any different exercise program and are a bit sore until they become accustomed to the movement. The muscles on the outside, inside and between your ribs will be sjretched. Even your shoulders, clavicles and shoulder blades, with all the muscles that are attached to them, must make adjustments; so you'll feel it.

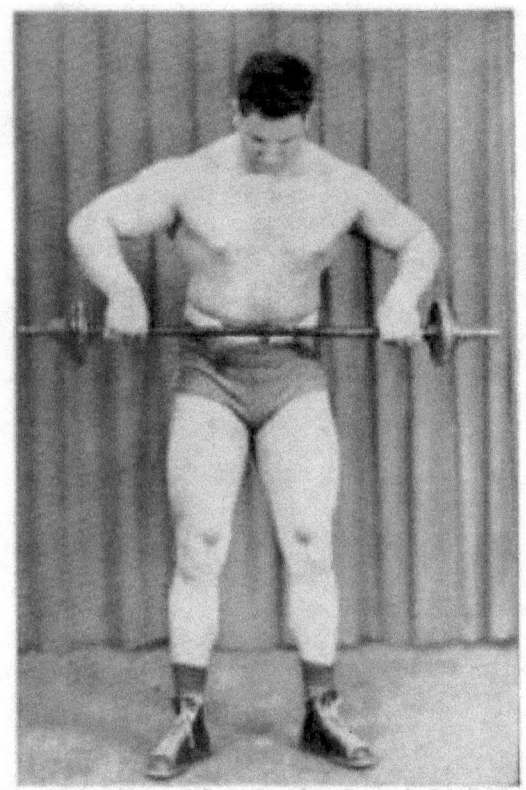

Big Dave Mayor, heavyweight lifting champion and America's strongest man of 1937. In this photo he weighs 263 pounds, has a 50-inch chest and a 19½-inch bicep. He weighed 4½ pounds as a baby, weighed 120 when he first reached his present height.

But don't mind that. Continue with your special training and you will be well rewarded in the end. Don't permit yourself to slump down during the day. Put into effect all the advice and instruction the chapter on posture contained; hold your chest up, not out; keep what you have gained.

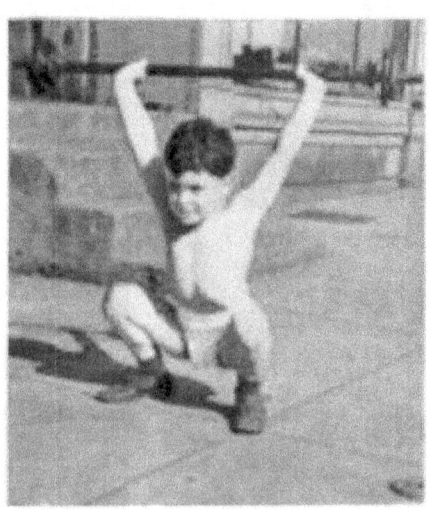

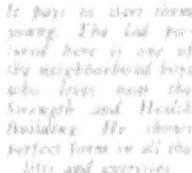

It pays to start them young. The lad forward here is one of the neighborhood boys who keeps most the Strength and Health Resolution. He shows perfect form in all the lifts and exercises.

After the completion of the twenty deep knee bends you should be breathless. That's what you want, and after a very short rest you should proceed to practice the pull over lying upon boxes or bench. This can be practiced upon the floor but it does not give you quite the range of movement. Unlike th" muscle building part of the two hands pull over, you need only a moderate weight. Many men were surprised to see Henry Steinborn, for long one of the world's strongest men, practicing this breathing exercise with a pair of fifteen-pound dumbells. A pair of twenties would not have been too great for Henry. I don't believe that any man should use more than fifty pounds in both hands. If you do use more than fifty, part of the value of the movement as a breathing exercise is lost. It then becomes a combination of only a fairly good breathing exercise and a poor muscle-building exercise. Better to practice the movement two ways—as a muscle builder for the latissimus and the pectorals of the cfiest, and with a moderate weight as a breathing exercise. To start you'll be wise to use not over thirty pounds unless you are accustomed to the movement and not more than forty pounds if you are in regular training. You can use a bar bell if you like or a pair of dumbells of the desired weight.

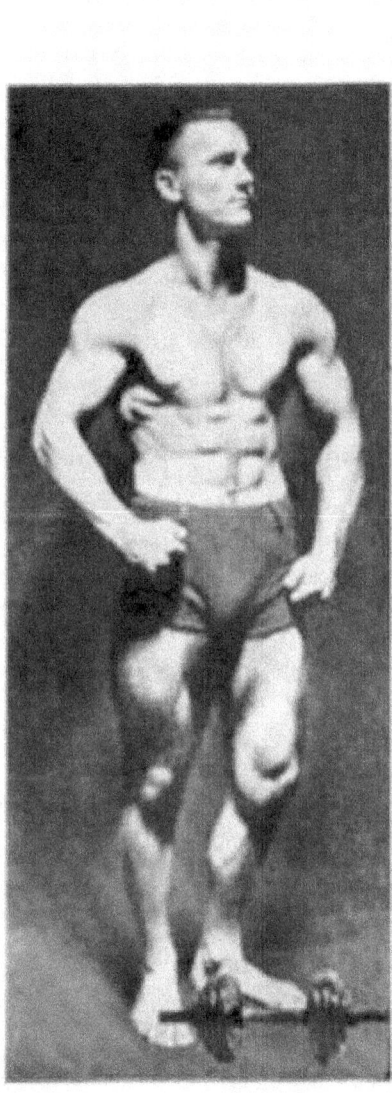

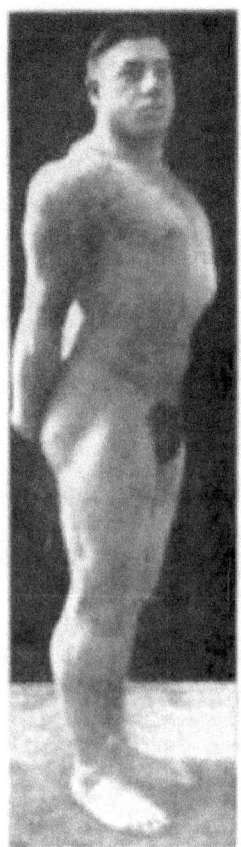

Jack Russell of London
Ontario, who for many
years was the best 148
pound lifter in the British
Empire, is shown here
weighing 767. Specializa-
tion on York dumbell training with comparatively
heavy weights, made it possible for him to gain over
15 pounds. Prior to this
special training he had
weighed 148 pounds for
years.

The usual procedure is practicing this movement when you
are not breathless and wish to develop muscles through it is
to move the bar bell or dumbells in a half circle from a

position back of head down to the thighs and back again. But in this strictly breathing exercise when you are already breathless and your internal parts are shouting for air and more air, you should move the arms only over a quarter circle. Lie down upon your back on the bench or boxes, press the bar bell or dumbells to arm's length overhead. In that position follow a system similar to that practiced with the deep knee bend—two deep breaths while the weight is held overhead, then with full lungs lower the bell behind the head; keeping arms straight, try to force even more air into the lungs. Widen and deepen the chest to the best of your ability. After the lowest position is reached, come back up again exhaling fully as the arms come to the directly overhead position. Two more full breaths and continue with the movement as described—twenty repetitions, forty breaths in all.

With these two movements which are a part of every York course you will have practiced one hundred deep breathing exercises. In specializing you will find it wise to perform both of these exercises two or three times. That means two hundred or three hundred deep breaths in all and you are sure to obtain good results. Many men who have reached a point in their training where they have failed to gain have discontinued all other forms of exercise for a month, have practiced this form of breathing exercise every day, and have gained four inches in chest size with this system. Upon the resumption of regular training they gained weight and muscle over their entire bodies at an astonishing rate.

This does not mean that the simple two exercise breathing course I have suggested is sufficient. It is better to practice it in conjunction with a complete exercise course or at least a few other good key exercises, such as press in front of or back of neck, rowing motion, press on box and the regular or stiff-legged deep knee bend. In the cases of men who have trained hard for a time and then ceased to gain, the change in the training course, more moderate and different work resulted in the rapid gains with the complete program. We recommend after a long period of intensive training that rest periods of from a week to two or more be experienced. These rest periods cannot be too frequent. This short course of specialization in breathing exercises is superior to a rest; it provides the change, yet gives the muscles a fair amount of work.

I like the press on boxes or bench as a breathing exercise. This is the one movement where one can breathe deeply while exercising with considerable weight. Regardless of how heavy the weight may be, it is possible to breathe fully and deeply in this exercise. If too much weight is utilized in the two hands pull over or even the deep knee bend or the stiff-legged dead weight lift, the breathing is restricted. In using the press on back as a muscle-building exercise select a weight which permits ten to twelve movements. It is beneficial in this way and a good combination exercise. It could be practiced with a somewhat lighter weight, more repetitions and deeper breathing, but the regular deep knee bend and the two hands pull over are as good as any, and you can use these to specialize in chest box increasing.

The stiff-legged dead weight lift lends itself well to the practice of breathing. Once again you must select a fairly light weight. Seldom more than body weight, not more than a hundred and fifty pounds, is best for most men. There are men who can practice this as a muscle-building exercise and use a very heavy weight without having a stiff back. Jack Cooper, Wally Zagurski and John Terry are three Yorkers who can use very heavy weights in this style. But there are others like myself who may feel a bit stiff in the spine after using a heavy weight in this manner. I have utilized up to three hundred pounds but always paid for it with a stiff back. So now I use only a moderate weight. My back is very flexible; in leaning back, for instance, with a

Roman chair, but it does not bend so well forward. This is an inherited quality and most men if they continue to strive for a form of flexibility for which they are not constructed will experience stiff backs.

For this type of man who has found it to be wise to use not more than a hundred and fifty pounds, there will be no temptation to handle too much weight. The other men must restrain themselves, using the movement as a breathing exercise as I am now suggesting. Practice this exercise as in the deep knee bend and the two arm pull over; three full breaths between movements, bending forward with full lungs, exhaling as you rise, then three full breaths.

In practicing these and other movements designed to increase the rib box, don't fail to breathe fully through the mouth three times at least between movements. Extend your ribs as much as possible in all exercises while breathing. Try to remain flat upon the bench while practicing the pull over. Don't permit the small of the back to rise. Work hard enough that you become breathless through the exercises and continue to breathe deeply as long after the completion of the exercise as possible. And remember to maintain good posture at all times while walking or sitting.

Using the pulleys which were constructed for latissimus development and recommended for the pectorals, breathing exercises are also possible. The latissimus movement where the arms are held straight overhead and then drawn to the side and down is the best breathing exercise with this equipment. Take your three breaths with the arms overhead, pull the arms down and exhale as you go up. This fine exercise will provide the dual purpose of building pectorals, latissimus and other muscles on the outside of the body while it expands the internal part of the chest.

It is easy to use a similar system with cable exercises, either the pull down from overhead or the press in front of or behind the back.

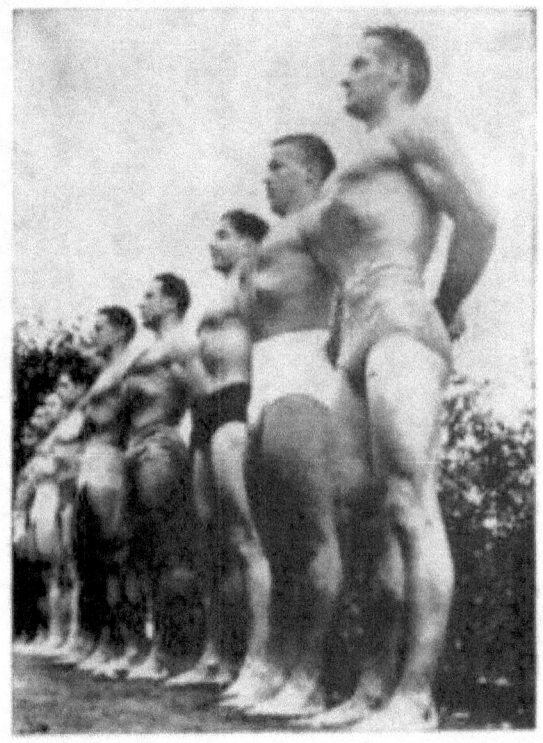

The Lapranos clan of Portland, Oregon, the strongest family in the world. While all are big, strong and well developed. Sam, fourth from the right, is most famed for his physique. He more closely approaches the Grecian physique than any man we have seen. There are six Lapranos here.
Cassel photo.

There are other good breathing exercises but I have offered the very best. They don't come any better and there is sufficient diversity of movement that you won't need any more. The important thing is to spend a goodly share of your training time at the proper practice of the deep breathing exercises I have recommended. And remember, please, that the important thing is not the amount of weight or resistance you use, but how you use it. Employ just enough to make you breathless.

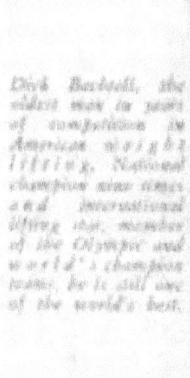

Dick Barbeell, the oldest man in years of competition in American weight lifting. National champion nine times and international lifting star, member of the Olympic and world's champion teams, he is still one of the world's best.

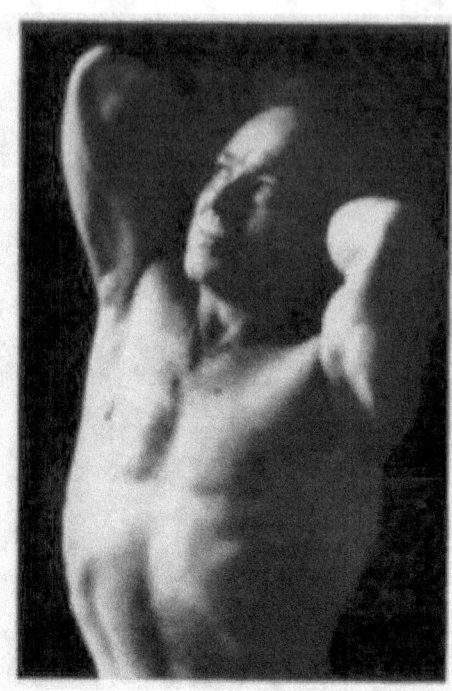

Displaying the Muscles of the Chest and Back

WHEN you have developed your rib box and the muscles which cover it to an advanced stage you should learn to isolate or control the various muscles and muscle groups and to display them to the best advantage. The muscles of the chest and back permit of many isolations and controls which when mastered will add to your appearance, your reputation as a strong, well-built man, and also can be the cause of much admiration, astonishment and hilarity when you illustrate your ability at muscle control before any group off riends or larger gathering.

It is debatable whether controlling your muscles will actually strengthen and develop them materially, but it is a fact that it will cause them to be clearer cut, and better appearing. You will be well rewarded in a variety of ways for the time and effort you expend in learning how to display or control your muscles.

All men, regardless of age, size or weight, have the same number of muscles and can learn to control them. But the undeveloped, " skinny" young man cannot offer a very pleasing display. The better built you are, the more pleasing will be your display and proportionately the more applause you will receive. Enthusiasts who gather at any strength show never tire of seeing the muscles displayed by as many stars of strength and development who are present as can be persuaded to offer an exhibition. At our big annual fall show which commemorates my birthday each year, practically every man who takes part in the program in any manner is persuaded to exhibit his muscles. The crowning feature of any show, of any strength exhibition, is the display of muscle control by that master of the art, the man who has won the titles, " world's best-built man," " world's most muscular man," and as this is written the holder of the official "Mr. America" title—Mr. John Grimek.

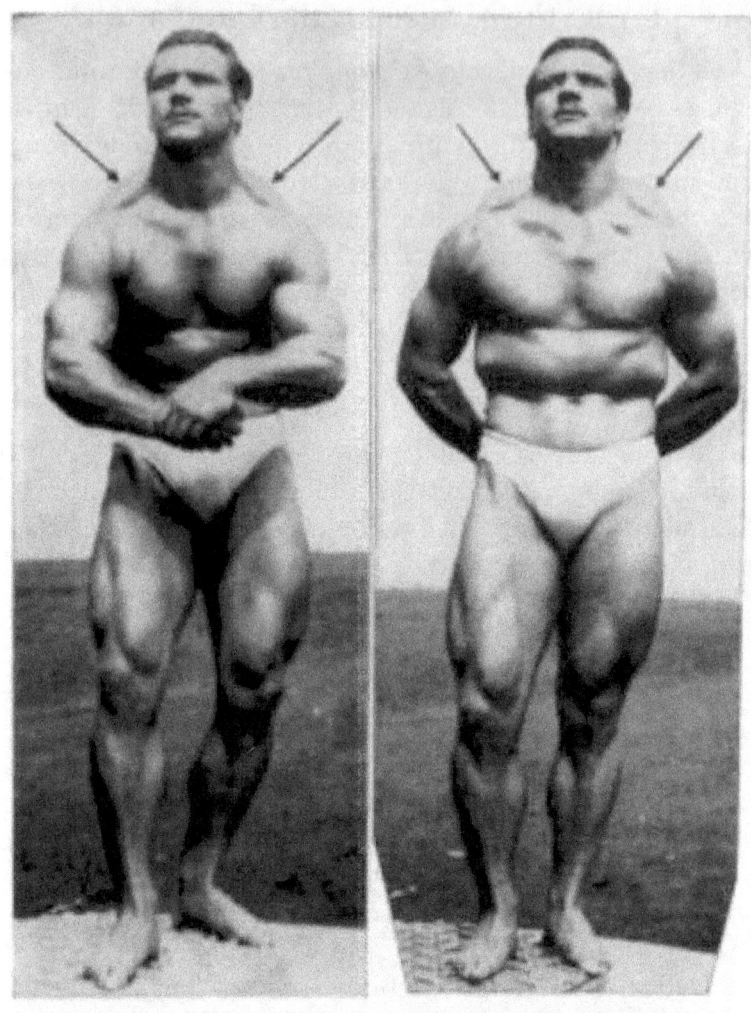

John Grimek, the master of muscle control.

Develop your muscles. Then become a master of the art of muscle control and success will be yours.

The pectorals or large muscles of the chest are easy to control and can be made to move in a startling manner. Although I have never offered a muscle control exhibition in my life, I can control most of my muscles, can shake a pencil out of my shirt pocket by wriggling my pectorals. In the beginning it is necessary to press the hands together to learn to control tljese muscles, but after a time you can shake or flick any of the muscles of the body without the assistance of the hands.

To begin, stand in front of a mirror; relax your muscles, especially the pectorals. Now press the hands against each other. You will notice that this slight exertion causes the pectorals to become rounded and tensed. Next learn to harden or tighten these muscles of the chest by flexing the muscles as the arms are folded across the chest. You will soon obtain control of these muscles and are ready to try more difficult controls.

To provide the most impressive display of these muscles assume the position illustrated by John Grimek. Here he is standing with the back a bit rounded, the shoulders bent forward, in an easy position to apply pressure to the hands, which makes it possible to jump the pectorals in an impressive manner. You can tense and relax the muscles successively and after a time will learn to control or separate the pectoralis major from minor which can be seen on John's photo where the arrow points to the hollow depression several inches below the clavicles or collarbones.

After you have learned to control these muscles readily, you can control them in a somewhat more advanced manner. Still standing with the back rounded and the shoulders forward, hold the hands out to the sides, and flick or control these muscles. In the beginning you can hold the hands out to supports at the side. Pull in on these supports, thus contracting the muscles. Soon you will learn to control them without any sort of outside help or pressure, although this feat is a great deal more difficult than when the hands are held together.

The advanced muscle control artist soon learns to control his pectorals while standing quite erect. With the arms at the sides, he tenses the pectoral muscles either simultaneously or alternately. As the movement continues they will seem to shake, wiggle or dance with great rapidity and usually someone will shout from the audience, "Who are you waving at?"

Absolute relaxation is the primary secret of all muscle control. Before the muscles are tensed as shown in the illustration by John Grimek, the muscles will be so loose that with a little tensing they will move or jump around. In each exhibition of muscle control, John Grimek illustrates that his muscies in repose are unusually soft and flexible. Many of those who are uninitiated concerning weight training think that weight lifters are muscle bound because they are always shown in photos with their muscles prominently displayed. Invariably, too, when you feel any of their muscles, they instantly tense them. Just try to catch any muscle man unaware and note that he instantly hardens his muscles when you touch him. While these muscles are rock-like when tensed, they are soft and pliable when in repose. The muscles of the strongest men are surprisingly soft when not tensed.

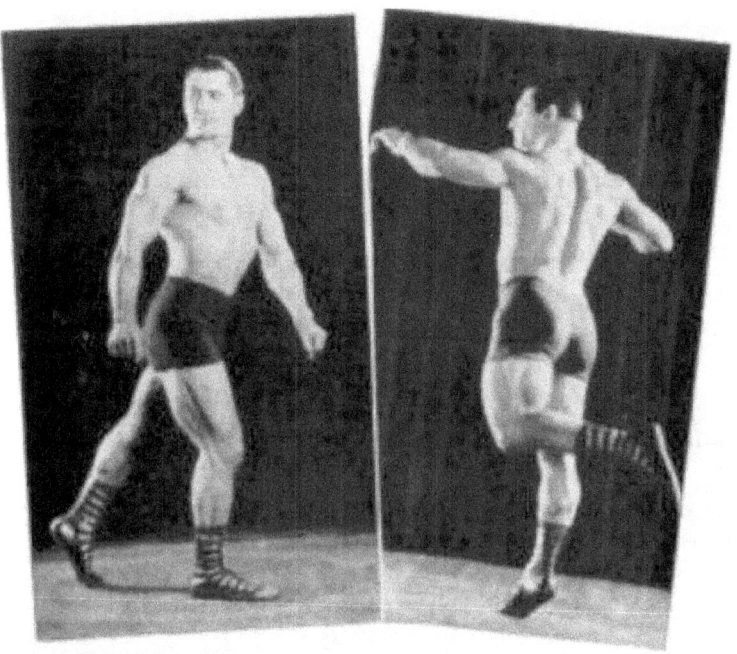

While the various abdominal controls should not be included in this book on the chest, they are the adjoining muscle group and you should learn to draw in the stomach by means of the vacuum and to perform an abdominal isolation. Briefly, this consists of leaning forward with hands on thighs, relaxing the muscles of the entire midsection and expelling the air from the lungs, which creates a vacuum and draws the muscles back to an astonishing degree. Then by tensing the muscles a rope is formed. I have seen young lads learn to perform this impressive feat in a few minutes, although it is a much harder task for a man of mature years. The serratus muscles which are commonly thought to be ribs can be displayed by any master of the art of muscle control. John Grimek has written several articles on muscle control which have appeared in Strength and Health magazine. These back copies can be had if you do not already have them.

The most impressive muscles of the back when displayed are the trapezius group. While these muscles which impart the slope to the shoulders of all strong men are most impressive in the star weight lifter, as they raise the shoulders, thus assisting in lifting the weight, the man who has done a reasonable amount, of bodybuilding with weights can learn to display these muscles to good advantage. The photo of John Grimek which was taken at our fall strength show illustrates an almost unbelievable degree of development and display of these muscles. One man wrote to us and said that he did not mind a little " touching up " of photos, but if we intended to " retouch " them in such an unbelievable manner, he would cease to purchase and read Strength and Health magazine. We assured him and all who see the photo that the photo and the negative are untouched, and we have them here to show to any who care to investigate. The cameraman was low, Grimek standing on a pedestal, and this did amplify the appearance of these muscles, but he being one of the strongest men in the world has a most unusual development of all the muscles and knows how to display them.

It is more difficult to learn to isolate the trapezius muscles than those of the pectorals, but if you persist your efforts will be rewarded. It is difficult to explain just how this muscle is isolated. With the partial description of the feat I can offer, and a close study of the photos, I believe you will learn something of how it is done. John Grimek explained that he first learned to control the muscle as follows: " Place hands behind back, interlacing the fingers, drawing the shoulders back and together, and then attempt to raise the arms, keeping them straight at the elbows throughout. As this is done you will note that two mounds of muscle will appear on top of the shoulders, along the neck. By this method it is impossible to isolate the trapezius to any great extent, but it will give you the " feel" of the muscle for better control of the muscle in other methods. Repeat this exercise several times and attempt to isolate the trapezius as indicated by the arrows in illustration number one and two. A different method is used in performing this isolation which I will presently explain.

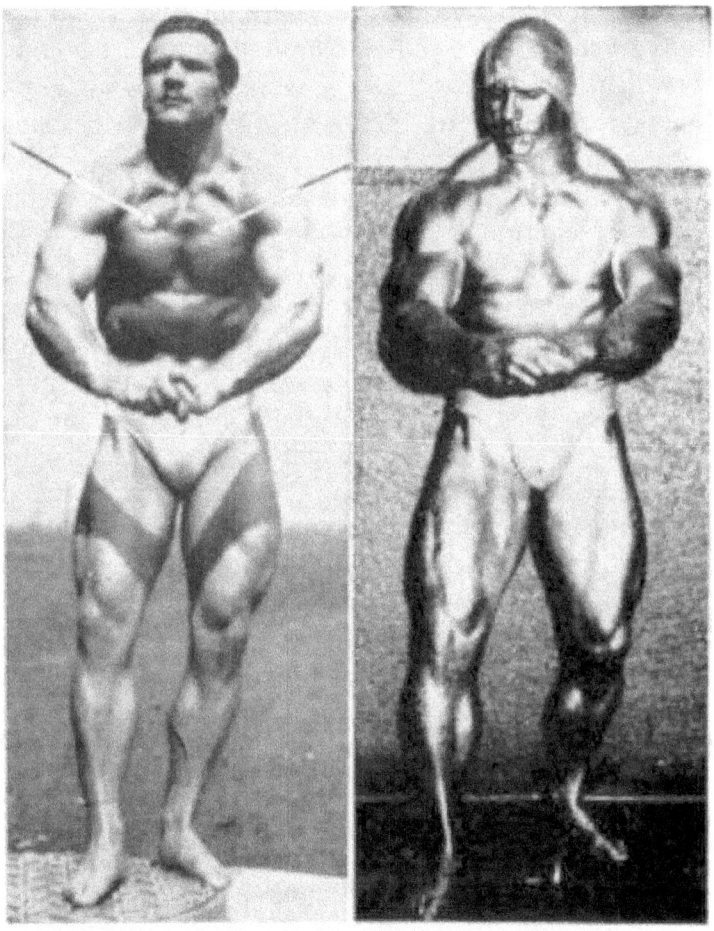

In the first figure Grimek is isolating the pectorals. Both the major and the minor can be clearly seen. In the second photo he is displaying the trapezius. It was this photo which caused some who had never actually seen John Grimek to believe that the photo had been retouched, but we can assure you that the picture is a true one of the Grimek physique. Neither the negative nor the print has been retouched or altered in any manner.

Figure five illustrates how the scapulae or shoulder blades 109k from the back when the trapezius is isolated, which can be done either single or double. You should spend considerable time in learning to control the shoulder blades for they are more impressive in action than most any muscle of the body. The double isolation is being shown in the picture. Assume a position before the mirror and clasp hands as shown in Figure 5. Preferably face the mirror rather than as in the side view which is shown for your convenience. I suggest that you first learn the single isolation, and, after you have learned that, then attempt the double. This should not be difficult when once you have learned to control a single scapulae. With your hands clasped as shown, drop one shoulder as low and as far forward as possible, and allow the shoulder to protrude as shown in the illustration. Press down with the other hand while resisting with the one on which you are trying to perform this isolation, keeping this arm almost straight at the elbow. The downward pressure will cause the scapulae to protrude to even a greater extent, also permitting the trapezius to become more prominent and isolated on top of the shoulders as shown in Figure 1. Always remember one thing when performing any trapezius controls: The latissimus dorsi muscles must be kept completely relaxed, and failure to do so will neutralize your efforts to display the trapezius. The anatomical construction of these muscles, both performing a different function, makes it relatively impossible to control them simultaneously. If you are having trouble isolating the trapezius look for your trouble in unconsciously tensing the latissimus. In nearly every case, failure to properly isolate the trapezius is the result of failure to properly and completely relax the latissimus.

In Figure i the trapezius is isolated in a manner similar to that shown in Figure 5. While these two figures show both the front and back views while the isolation is in progress it should give you a good idea of how the isolation is performed. In Figure 1 the shoulders are brought forward and the pressure is exerted in an attempt to break open the grip, allowing the scapulae to dislocate as shown in Figure 5, resulting in the isolation as indicated by the arrows in Figure 1.

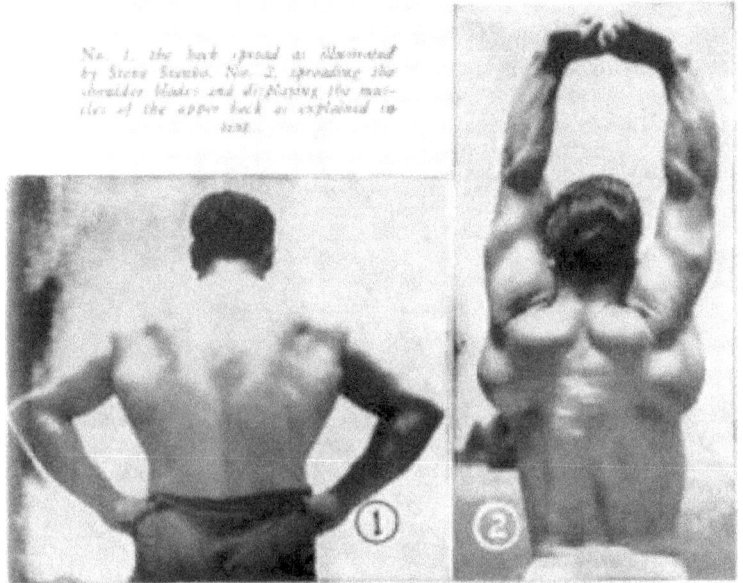

No. 1. the back spread as illustrated by Steve Stanko. No. 2. spreading the shoulder blades and displaying the muscles of the upper back as explained in text.

After you have learned the isolation of the trapezius, you will find that the method shown in Figure 2 is one of the easiest ways to control the trapezius and you will be able to isolate them in this manner far easier than in any other way. You place your hands on the small of your back, on your hips as shown in Figure 2, leaning your shoulders slightly forward in this position. By pressing with the back of your hands against your back and at the same time down, the scapulae will isolate and protrude from the back as shown in Figure 5. The large trapezius muscles beside the neck will be prominently isolated as indicated by the arrows in the photograph. This isolation can be done either singly or doubly, but it is more impressive and comical when performed alternately.

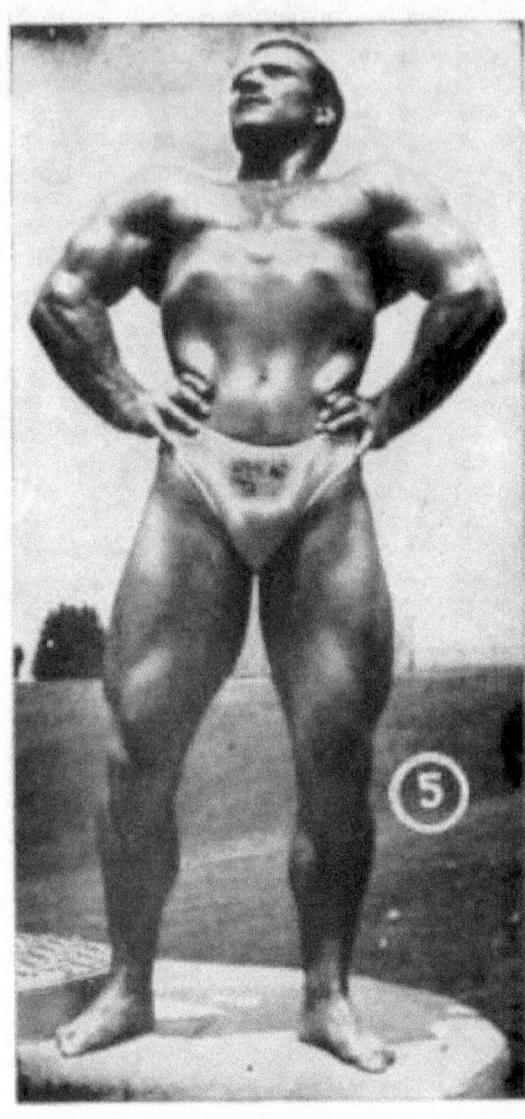

Fig. 3. A remarkable picture of John Grimek, spreading the shoulder blades and widening the Latissimus.

Big-Chested Men

I HAVE before me a list of 158 men past and present who are or have been prominent in the strength world. It would be wonderful if these measurements could have been taken with the same tape, by the same man, while each athlete was at his best. Then we would have an actual comparison. While it is more than possible that some of the chest measurements contained in the statistics of these 158 men on my list are exaggerated a bit, it is just as likely that many of them did not obtain the best measurement of which they are capable. To obtain this list, I have delved deep in most of the books in my library, and have searched through every issue of Strength and Health magazine from its inception in 1932.

Some of the measurements are given as normal, others as expanded. There is such a great difference in the conception of a normal chest (for instance men like Arthur Saxon, who cared nothing for measurements, could easily enough have been standing in his habitually careless, slouching position when the measurements were taken). His chest size of 48 inches, while large for a man of 5 feet, 10 inches, weight 210, does not seem to be the best of which he was capable. His great bent pressing ability must have given him exceptional latissimus dorsi development and had he expanded this to the limit, I believe that the tape would have been stretched to a full 50 inches.

George Hackenschmidt gained fame as having the largest chest of any athlete of his time. He has been credited with a chest of 52 inches at one stage of his career. However, in his own book, "The Way to Live," I find that at the age of nineteen, when he weighed 176 at his height of 5 feet, 8 1/2 inches, his chest was 46 expanded. Two years later, when he was bigger and much stronger and was making world weight lifting history, his weight had increased. to 196 and his chest to 47 Later in his career he weighed somewhat more, but one would hardly-expect a chest gain of nearly five inches, with this slight increase of body weight, particularly when Hackenschmidt himself insisted that he did not train with bar bells after 1908, during which year he was world's wrestling and weight lifting champion. A photo of him was shown some years ago in an English magazine, in which his chest was most impressive and definitely huge in size. I met him personally two years ago when he visited this country. He weighed about the same as he did in 1908, and although he was a powerfully constructed, heavy-boned man, he was strong, heavy and well- developed all over and it did not seem to me that he would have had at any stage of his career a chest of more than 50 inches. I hope I am not detracting from the reputation of this great old timer. I am sure that Hackenschmidt himself would put us right on this question of his chest size if we had the opportunity to ask him, for he is very honest in everything that concerns his lifting and other athletic records. Judging that his chest is not over 50 inches, I take into consideration that his build is quite similar to Steve Stanko's, the present world's and United States heavyweight lifting champion, yet he is 25 pounds lighter in weight, and shorter in height, and Steve's very well developed, deep, rounded, fine-appearing chest barely places him in the 50-inch class. Therefore I should think that if we credit George Hackenschmidt with a 50-inch chest we are being fair with him.

There was a wide difference in all his measurements as offered by Eugene Sandow. In his book, published in 1894, " Life is Movement," he reported his own expanded chest size at 60 inches. Later in the book he included his measurements as taken by famous Dr. Sargent of Harvard University and the chest circumference is 46 inches. Sandow weighed 180, his height was 5-8, and a chest of 46 inches is good-sized for such a height and weight. It is reasonable to believe that Sandow's actual chest measurement was 46 inches and not the 60 inches he reported.

The biggest chest we have on record was the property of Louis Cyr, the Great French-Canadian strong man, generally believed to have been the strongest man who ever lived. His weight fluctuated from 275 to 315, so there would be a difference in chest measurement at these varying weights. His measurements as offered in the book, " The Strongest Man Who Ever Lived," are 59 1/2 at one stage of his career and 60 inches at another. It is reasonable to believe that these" measurements are accurate, for Louis was 5 feet 10 inches in height—2 inches more than that of the normal man—yet he was so huge, deep and round that he looked very short. He was built in proportion, having a biceps and calf of over 20 inches.

Another giant of strength, often considered to have been as strong or even stronger than Cyr, was Louis Uni, best known as Appolon. He was a Frenchman, and is credited with a normal chest of 50 inches at a height of 6-3, and a body weight of 265 pounds. Many authorities in the strength world have ranked Appolon and Cyr as the two strongest men of recorded history. Appolon's measurements were extraordinary as far as the other parts of his body were concerned. He is credited with a biceps of 20 inches, a straight forearm of 17 1/2, flexed 19, 30-inch thigh, 20 1/2-inch calf. It is reasonable to believe that he would have had a chest measurement expanded of not less than 52 inches, in consideration of the marvelous measurements of other parts of his body.

Herman Gorner, the German from South Africa, is claimed by some to have been the strongest man in the world. He has left some truly extraordinary records behind him. He was a tall man, height 6 feet, 1 inch, somewhat slender in the legs, yet 245 pounds in body weight. His measurements were given to us by his trainer, Tromp Von Diggelen, as 46 inches normal chest and 52 1/2 inches expanded. It is rare for a strong man to have much variation between normal and expanded chest, and it is possible that Gorner's conception of a normal chest was quite deflated. His strength, size and weight were such that his measurement of 52 inches expanded chest is what we would expect. Gorner ranks near the head of the list among big-chested men.

Henry Steinborn ranks among the old timers in point of experience and reputation. Forty-seven years of age at present, he is still active and considered to be the strongest man in professional wrestling. While a young man, a bit after the great war of 1914-18, he came to this country and immediately set a number of world's weight lifting records, and was freely considered to be the strongest man in the world of the time. He was not a huge man when compared with some of the great strong men we have been discussing; he weighed 210 in 1920, the same weight as Arthur Saxon in his prime, and he was approximately the same height. In the photo in which he appears with the writer of this

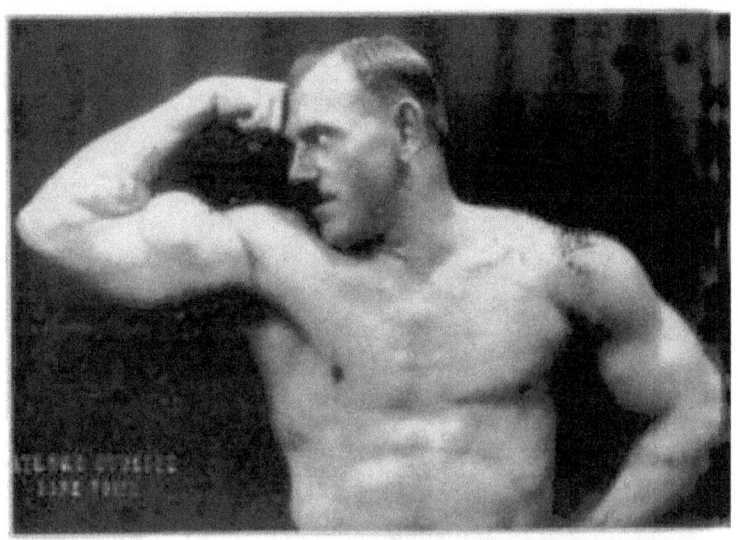

Herman Gorner, the South African German. One of the strongest men who ever lived.

Clevio Massimo is about fifty years of age as this is written. In 1933 I believe he was the most muscular man I ever saw. John Grimek, the most muscular man in the world at present, has somewhat better proportions, but for sheer, rock-like, rugged power and appearance of his muscles it is doubtful if Massimo at his best has ever been excelled. Massimo was 5 feet 8 1/22 inches, exactly John Grimek's height; he weighed 194, very close to John's weight which fluctuates as he desires—as low as 181 for championship lifting (he weighed 183 the day he won the Mr. America title and the additional titles, " Most Muscular Man in America," and "America's Best-Built Man") and he weighs 200 pounds at times. While these official titles include only America, there is no other man in the world who closely rivals him for development and beauty of physique. Massimo had a 46-inch normal chest and probably it would have been at least 48 inches expanded—not quite as large as the Grimek chest, but with the same weight and height, and not the same narrowness of waist, it is natural that

Grimek would excel in chest measurement to make up for the wasp-like slenderness of his waist.

Joe Nordquest was one of the greatest of American strong men. While handicapped by the loss of a lower limb in childhood, he became strong enough to break world's weight lifting records. He is credited with a chest of 47 1/2 inches. Warren Lincoln Travis, dean of strong men who are still active, is a big powerful man who excels at back and harness lifting. Powerfully built in the lower limbs, he is also barrel like in chest construction. Some of his best records were made at a body weight of 185, but at the present he weighs over 200 and is credited with a chest of 48 inches.

The very largest of the chests of the old time strong men of which we have a record have been mentioned, but our statistics of big-chested men would not be complete unless we mention two smaller men, men who are very big-chested in proportion to their size and weight. The first of these is my friend Oscar Matthes of Lawrence, Mass., a man who is seventy-eight years of age as this is written and still a strong man. In his prime he weighed from 105 to 108 pounds. His height was 4 feet 10 inches and his bodily measurements were as near perfection as those of any man. He attained what had been considered to be the ideal measurements, the most hoped-for measurements for a man of his bony framework and short stature. His chest of 40 inches, coupled with a waist of 28 inches, was truly impressive. His personal friend and for many years training mate, John Y. Smith, a great old time strong man of New England, now seventy-six years of age, had all the chest one could expect for a man of his size and body weight, at 44 inches normal. He weighed but 160 at the time, the same body weight which carried him when he won the title, " Strongest Man in All New England "—a triumph which he won when he was sixty years of age. His chest should have been an inch or two larger expanded, and that would have been most extraordinary for a man of his wiry frame and only 160 pounds in body weight.

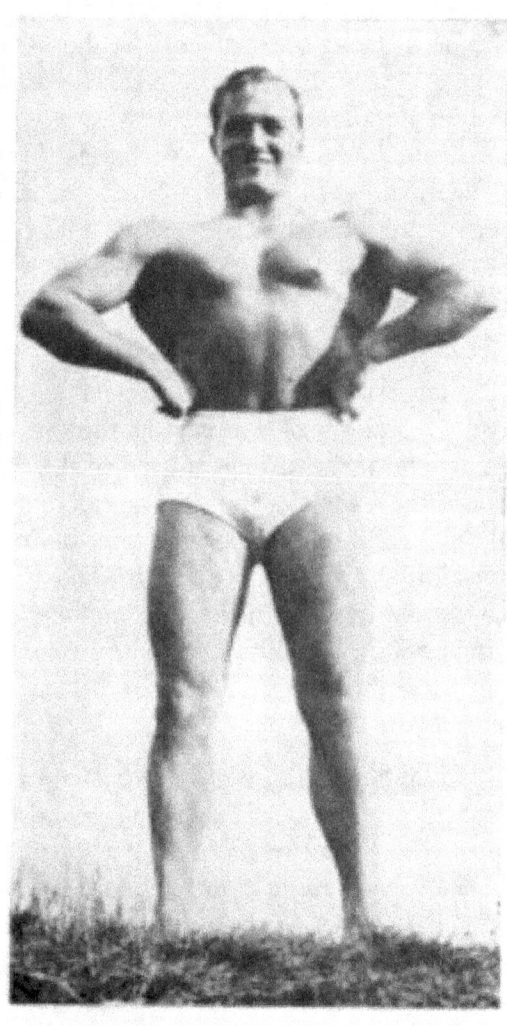

Joe Peters, of Schenectady, N. Y., displaying his 53-inch chest and 31-inch waist, the greatest differential in chest and waist measurement of which we have a record.

Of the newer generation of strong men, Joe Peters, son of the chief of police in Schenectady, N. Y., and now a patrolman, has the best chest. In addition to having the greatest size—53 inches—he has the greatest differential between chest and waist size—waist 32 inches, chest 53, a difference of 21 inches. While not a competitive lifter, he is a very strong young man and excels at many strength feats for which he has received numerous awards. He won the award, " Best Developed Chest," at the Mr. America Contest of 1939, at Amsterdam, N. Y. His closest competitor was Walter Podolak, now a professional wrestler, formerly world's record holder in the two hands dead weight lift at which he made a record of 643. Podolak does not have nearly as large a chest as Joe Peters, for he is only 5 feet 6 inches in height, but it is extremely large and broad in proportion to his size. Forty-eight inches on his smaller body looks as impressive as the 53-inch Joe Peters' chest.

The next largest chest of which we have a record is that of Gregory George, best known as the St. Louis Samson. George is one of the strongest men in the world at present. He weighed 325 as a boy of sixteen. Weight training brought his weight to a much trimmer build of 260 pounds. He is a similar type to Louis Cyr. The first time he ever lifted a weight he dead lifted 600 pounds and performed a deep knee bend with 400. At the time he competed in the national championships in weight lifting he had a chest measurement of 52 inches.

Peters and George are the only two men of whom I have a record, aside from myself, who have chests of 52 inches. My chest equals that of George in measurement, but I am taller—six inches more—and it would not look as huge. My chest has grown from 36 inches, when I returned from France after the last war, to its present 52 inches. Although a big man may not look as terrifically developed as some shorter men, the very fact that he is big results in large measurements. John Grimek at his body weight of 200 seems to be a fair-sized man, but he is small when compared with Stanko or myself. When he tried on my new coat which fitted me very well, it hung almost like a sack upon him. And certainly my physique does not even compare in proportions or development with Grimek's.

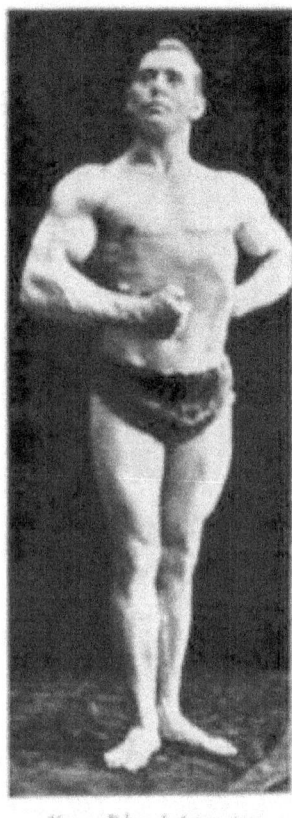

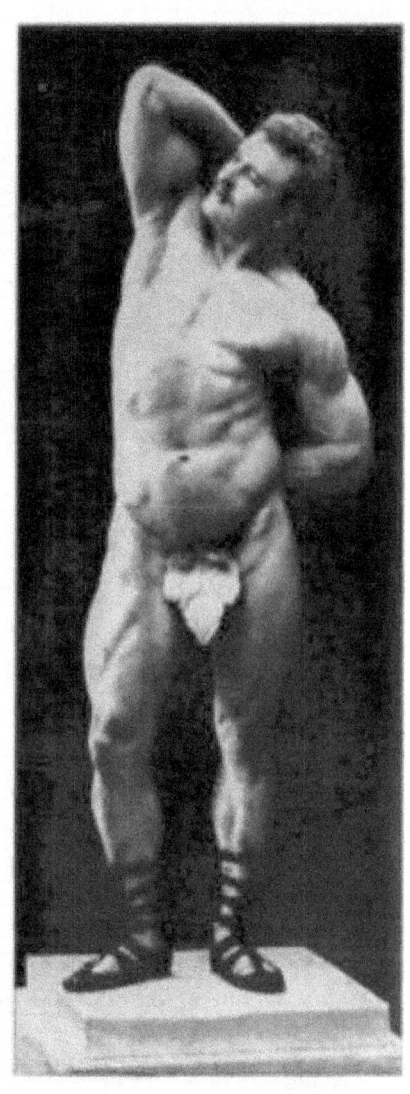

Above: Edward Aston, formerly Britain's strongest man. Although he weighed only 168 he possessed phenomenal strength.

Eugene Sandow, the most famous strong man in history.

At the Mr. America contest this year, Frank Leight, the New York policeman whose real name is Stepenak, won the best-developed chest award. Frank has a magnificent body, one of the best in the world. He's a big man too, weighing around 210. The only actual measurement I have of him is 47 1/4 inches chest normal. Surely his fine, deep chest would measure at least 50 inches expanded. Louis Abele, another young giant, continues to grow both in strength and development and has now reached the 50-inch class. Louis weighs 220 at present and as he is still growing should have a chest one of these days which rivals that of Joe Peters.

Everett Marshall, the wrestler, ranks with the biggest-chested men. He's just average height—5-8—but weighing 226, as he does, he has a splendid chest—49 inches normal and 51 inches expanded. He is an unusual athlete; can chin himself 28 times; also chins with one hand, which is splendid for a big man.

Other men with 50-inch chests are John Grimek, Steve Stanko, Frank Jares, the Pacific Coast heavyweight lifting champion, Dave Mayor, heavyweight champion of 1937, that year America's strongest man, body weight 265, with an arm of 19 inches, and Jake Hitchins, a young man from Carlisle, Pa., who excels at the flying exercise, employing up to 100 pounds in this exercise.

In the 49-inch class we have Weldon Bullock and Chick Deutch; at 48 inches, Jack Lalanne, of Oakland, Cal. (Jack is not a big man, probably not weighing more than 170, but he has extraordinary development of pectorals, upper back muscles and latissimus dorsi which gives him one of the world's finest chests); Bert Goodrich, all-around athlete, member of the hand balancing team of Goodrich and Nelson, one of the best in the business, the winner of the Amsterdam, N. Y., Perfect Man Contest of 1939; Bill Panzen, wrestler and weight lifter, body weight 210; Gord Venables of the York Bar Bell Club, and Jack Cooper, 6 feet 4 y_2 inches, nineteen-year-old star lifter of the same club.

I will list a few other big-chested men—Joe Miller whose chest grew from 32 to 42 one year later when he was eighteen years of age (Joe, you may remember, was one of the original members of the York team, one of the strongest men in the world, and 181-pound champion of 1936 and a member of the Olympic team of that year); Ray Van Cleef, famous physical culturist and writer for Strength and Health magazine, has a 46-inch expanded chest; Joe Raymond, a man who built his weight from 133 to a full 200 pounds, weight lifting chairman in the Ohio district, a 46-inch chest; Tony Petroline, the Chicago weight lifter who formerly weighed 200 pounds, reduced to a splendid and powerful physique of 160 and became one of the best middleweight lifters in the nation (in fact later, lifting overweight, he tied with Gord Venables for second place in the national championships of 1936, 181-pound class), has a 47-inch expanded chest; George Kiehl, one of the finest before and after cases of which we have a record, built his weight in stages from 120 to 186, ended with one of the finest physiques in the land and an expanded chest of 46 1/2 inches; Jack Channing, of the Pittsburgh Central Y. M. C. A., a winner of several best-built man contests, and one of the famous York Bar Bell men, has a chest of 46 inches; Emil Bonnet, one of our very good friends, a man who trained with Siegmund Klein and later won the best- built man contest in France, has a 46 1/2-inch normal chest at his height of 5 feet 11 1/2 inches and weight of 185; Sam Loprinzi of the Multnomah A. C., Portland, Ore., the man who has a physique which is nearer to that of John Grimek than any we have seen is 5 feet 7 inches, weighs 170 pounds and has a 47-inch chest; Jesse James, world's light-heavyweight wrestling champion, one of our famous York Bar Bell men, weighs 175 and has a fine-appearing 46-inch chest; Ben Markley, former weight lifting champion of the South Atlantic district, a member of the Baltimore, Md., fire department, is 5 feet 9 inches, weighs 185 and has a 47-inch chest.

Roger Eells, the man who overcame an advanced case of tuberculosis and increased his body weight from 121 to 200, has a 47y$_2$-inch chest. John Terlazzo, brother of our famous world champion Anthony Terlazzo, one of the best middleweight lifters in the nation, is 5 feet 7 inches, weighs 170 and has a 45-inch chest. John Gallagher, a light-boned man of 186 pounds who won the Great 1940 Strength and Health Self-Improvement Contest from among over 6000 official entries, is 5 feet 9 inches and has a 47-inch chest. Barton Horvath, long famed as the possessor of one of the world's best physiques, a good light-heavyweight lifter, 5 feet 8 inches in height, has a chest of 46 inches.

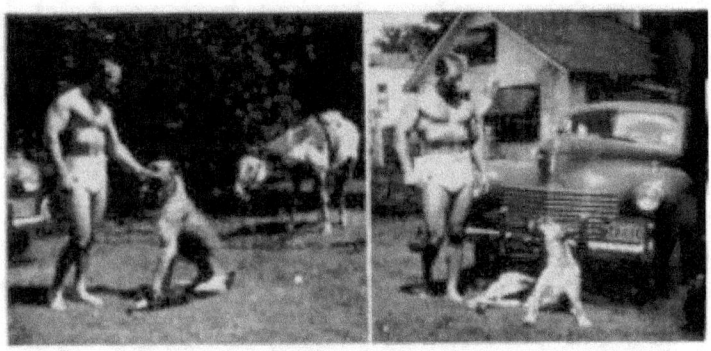

George Gallagher, of the Paterson A. C., Bergenst, N. J., winner of the Great Strength and Health Self-Improvement Contest. These photos taken the day he arrived in York. His bodyweight is 186, he having gained 18 pounds from his already powerful physique during the contest.

Among our own men of the York Bar Bell Club, John Grimek and Steve Stanko with their 50-inch chests lead the list. Gord Venables is next with 48. Then come John Davis and Jack Cooper with 47—this measurement of Jack Cooper at 212 and 6 feet 4 inches, of John Davis at 195; at times he weighs more and then his chest is larger. His chest is very impressive and very likely in a moderate period of time will reach 50 inches. Wally Zagurski, 5 feet 6 1/2 inches in height, 180 pounds in body weight, has a 47- inch chest. John Terpak and Eddie Harrison measure 441/2. John weighs 165 and is 5 feet 6 inches in height, Eddie 5 feet inches and a bit over 150. Tony Terlazzo, height 5 feet 4 inches, has a truly magnificent chest for a man of such moderate height with his circumference of 44 inches.

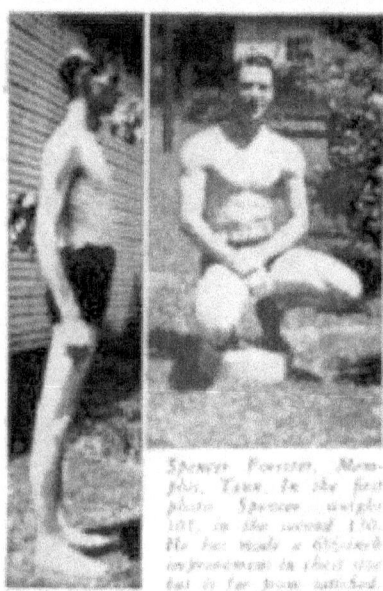

Spencer Forester, Memphis, Tenn. In the first photo Spencer weighs 103, in the second 130. He has made a distinct improvement as these two but is far from satisfied.

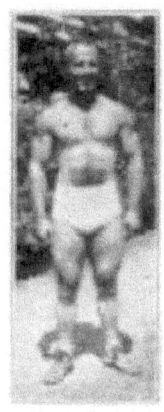

Art Levan, of the York Bar Bell Club, as the time he was in the midst of winning his astonishing string of 10 consecutive 126-pound United States championships. Photo taken at the Olympics of 1932 in California.

Art Levan, two inches less in stature, national 126-pound champion for ten consecutive years, now weighs 145, and is a miniature Hercules. His chest measurement is 42. John Terry, national 132-pound champion, and world's record holder in the dead weight lift with a record of 610, is 5 feet inches and has a chest of 40 inches. He has one of the world's most powerful and best-developed physiques. He's definitely the strongest man of his pounds in the world, and his well-moulded, good-sized chest with a tapering, slender waistline creates a most pleasing effect. Dick Bachtell, national 132-pound champion nine times, the oldest man in point of years of service in competitive weight lifting, is 5 feet 2 inches, weight 135 and has a chest of 40 inches.

This chapter contains sufficient of statistics to give you an idea who had the largest chest among the greats of the past, who ranks at the head of the men of today, and just what you can expect from your height and bone framework.

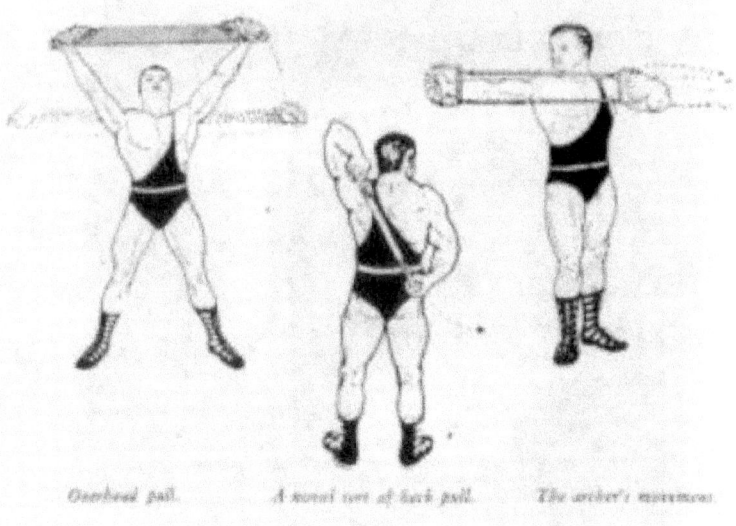

Overhead pull.   A novel sort of back pull.   The archer's movement.

More Important Chest Facts

THERE IS a vast difference in methods of measuring the chest, just as there was confusion in measuring the arm until we endeavored to clarify the methods of measurement with our three positions. Arm size of heavyweight prize fighters was always relatively small and few could understand how these men who weighed at least two hundred pounds could have only thirteen- and fourteen-inch arms. Considerable perplexity arose. Now the well-informed body builders explain that their arms are such a size in the No. 1, No. 2 or No. 3 position and equally well-informed readers will be familiar with these designations and therefore it will be much easier to make comparisons.

Chest measurements are sent in with every report and every success story. They are usually offered normal, and expanded. To take the normal measurement you should stand at ease with the chest neither deflated nor expanded, as near normal as it can be held in a quiescent state. Some men are of the opinion that normal chest means contracted and thus they manage to obtain an apparent greater expansion in inches. Be sure that you do not tense the pectorals or the muscles of the side or back in taking this normal measurement. It is easier to have someone else take your measurements to be sure that the tape is not sloped, but if you are entirely alone take the measurement in front of a mirror so that you can see the position of the chest.

The measurement should always be taken in the same position. Hold the tape firmly against the body but do not tighten it unnecessarily, cutting into the flesh. Tapes that are employed for long periods have a tendency to shrink, particularly when used while you are perspiring and this may falsely cause you to believe that you are gaining more rapidly than you truly are. Obtain a metal tape if it is convenient. The tape should be placed either directly over the nipples or a trifle above them; it should go right around the body under the armpits.

It will add to the ease of measuring your chest if you will obtain a tape with a metal ring on the end. Otherwise you will feel that you should have at least three hands, or eyes in the back of your head. The important thing in obtaining an accurate measurement is to keep the tape level. Handling the tape yourself causes a tendency to make it slip down in the back and to raise it over the breastbone or sternum in the front, causing the tape to pass around your body at an angle and unfairly exaggerating the size of your chest.

Standing at ease in preparation for taking the normal chest measurement, the right arm will hang at the side, holding the free end of the tape with the left hand. If you are taking the measurements to send with your enrollment blank it is particularly important that proper measurements be sent so that a false idea of your starting condition or resulting gains is not obtained.

Men who exult in their strength and muscles take pride in their chest expansion and chest size too and it is very difficult for such men to take an accurate, normal chest measurement. This type of man will force all the air out of his lungs and pull the tape so tight it cuts into his flesh. But this is not the measurement of the normal chest; it is the measurement of thq contracted chest. As cited in an earlier chapter, if you stand erect, without the lungs inflated however, you will have a sizeable normal chest, and not a very great chest expansion. From contracted measurements to full expansion this man may claim five to seven inches, thinking that he is not as strong a man as others who claim a big expansion. Yet his normal expansion should be only from one to three inches if the measurement of the chest actually normal is taken.

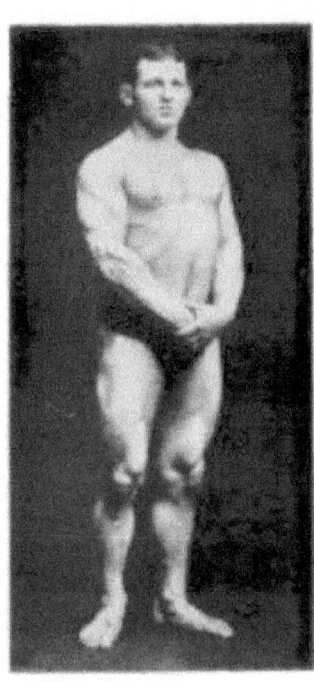

John Lemm, mountain guide of the Swiss Alps. Possessor of one of the finest physiques in the world

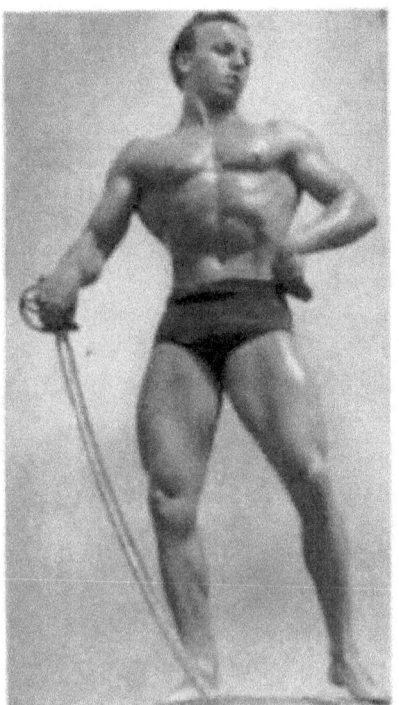

Leonard Schafer, of the Passaic, N. J., Y. M. C. A., a leader in the bar bell movement at that organization

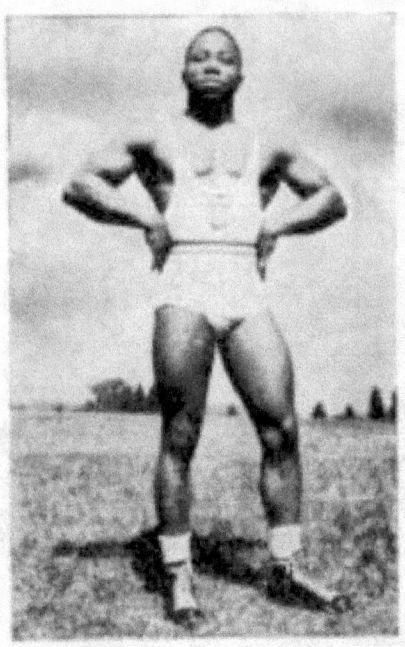

To obtain the proper measurement of the expanded chest, keep the tape in the position in which you measured your normal chest. Inhale as much as you are able, forcing out the ribs as far as you can from pressure of your expanding lungs. When you have reached the limit of your expansion read the tape measure. Don't flex your muscles in obtaining this measurement for you wish to know the actual size of your rib box so that you can properly measure your gains in the future. You can tense your muscles front, back and sides now to see how great a measurement you can obtain with lungs filled to the limit and muscles tensed. You can keep a record of three chest measurements:

1.   Contracted.

2.   Normal.

3.   Expanded—muscles tensed and expanded to their limit.

You could obtain the lung expansion better by measuring below the pectorals but it has been customary to measure the chest around the pectorals and only confusion will result if we recommend another position.

In trying to obtain superexpansion of the chest, with the greatest range between contracted and fully expanded chest, you should first of all hunch the shoulders, pressing them slightly forward, and flattening your chest in an endeavor to make your thorax or rib box as small as possible. From this position come erect, holding the chest as high as possible, the shoulders back, the rib box inflated to its limit, the back spread as far as possible and the chest muscles hardened.

Practice in front of a mirror will aid you in becoming so skilled at muscle control that you can obtain your maximum measurement. Drawing in the waist amplifies the appearance of size of the chest. If you are posing with your front toward the camera, only width of your chest will be displayed, but if you are posing sideways or partly so, a well-distended chest will show to particular advantage.

There are few professionals on the stage at present, although a number of them are still making the rounds of the county fairs. Exhibitions of chest expansions are at times shown, particularly with the chain breaking feat previously described. Some of these men have used one and even two derby hats under their belt, removed them and filled the belt with chest and muscle expansion. Only the biggest chested men could duplicate the feat of Arthur Dan- durand of Montreal. Dandurand is still living, about sixty years of age at present, and still most remarkable. He is a light-boned man, one of the handful of men in the history of muscle culture who officially exhibited a measurement of forearm which was more than twice that of wrist when the arm is held straight. With these light bones he developed splendid muscular proportions and a slender waist which was offset most impressively by his huge chest. He would have an assistant stand inside a strap placed around his chest, and when the assistant had wormed his way from under the belt he would expand until the strap was filled. It would be impressive for any of you who wish to put on a good act to include this in your performance. The assistant should stand in front of you so that his body and one arm are within the belt. The belt should first of all be placed around your abdomen, then raised a bit, and particularly with an assistant smaller than you no one can determine that the belt is around the largest part of the chests of both. When the assistant has escaped, raise the belt around the largest part of your body and fill it. This feat and the breaking of chains should be of material benefit in aiding you to establish a record and reputation as a strong man in your part of the country.

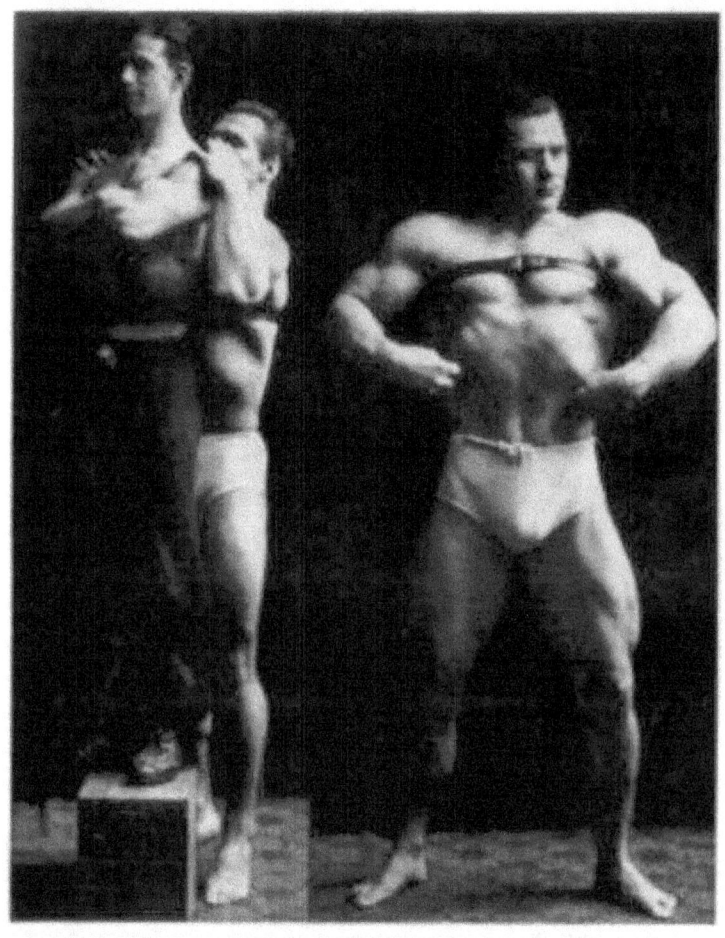

Another good feat is to take a truck tire inner tube, remove the valve stem and learn to inflate this tube simply by the constant pressure from your own lungs. I saw a professional, who had formerly been tubercular, performing this feat at each act. He would continue until the tube would burst. There is always a weak spot in a tube which will be forced out into a big lump before the remainder of the tube and that is where the break would take place.

Some men unfortunately have defects in their chests which are difficult to overcome. Some describe their difficulty as a hole in their chest, a very definite depression; others are pigeon or chicken breasted. This was my difficulty originally. At first glance it would seem that the sternum protrudes as it does in a bird, causing this condition of chicken breast. But usually the breastbone is in a normal position; the ribs are deflated. In this latter case the condition can be overcome by expanding the chest to an extent that the ribs flare out a great deal more. An improvement of the pectoral muscles will benefit this condition from the standpoint of actual appearance and development.

While pigeon or chicken breast is fairly common, the condition of flat chest is much more prevalent. It is usually accompanied by what we know as round shoulders. For, more than any other one thing, poor posture which has compressed the chest has caused it to be flat in appearance. Flat chest is really shallow chest and it comes about through lack of development and poor posture. When the chest is flat in the front from early childhood in order to have more room in the rib box, the shoulder blades are extended to the rear and the condition of round shoulders is increased. There must be room in the chest cavity for the proper operation of the heart and lungs so the shoulder blades are pushed out in the back in a natural condition of flat or shallow chest.

It is possible to become strong while permitting your body to be in this position. I have seen gymnasts, who specialized in dipping, and wrestlers, who had developed the crushing muscles of their chest and arms while neglecting the back, who had this flat-chested, round-shouldered appearance yet were very well-developed otherwise. Too much emphasis on pectoral development without sufficient of upper back exercise to counterbalance it will produce this condition of flat chest and round shoulders. If there is sufficient room for the organs, as a result of constant training, the man will not be unhealthy, but certainly he won't present a very admirable appearance.

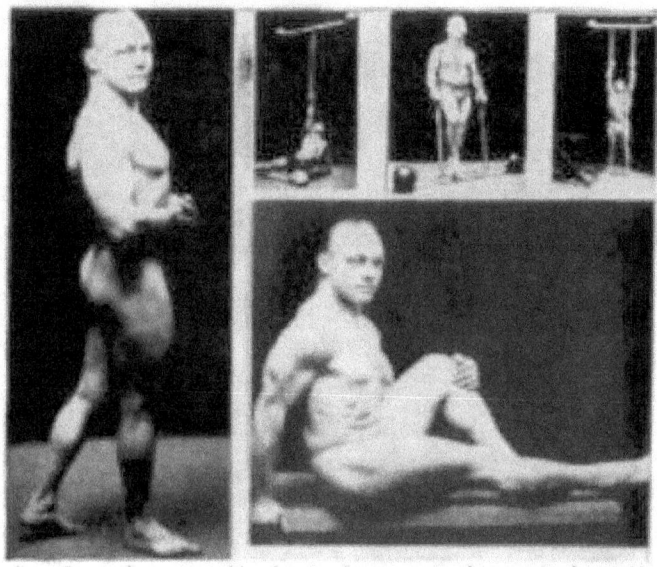

Otto Arco, who was considered to be the most muscular man in the world while he was active professionally. He had the largest arm on record for body weight, 17¼ inches, bodyweight 134, a chest of 43 inches, and was one of the first three men in the world to jerk double his bodyweight overhead. He toured the world and he and his brother were one of the highest paid acts in vaudeville. One look at his back served under the lights brought more spontaneous applause than most athletes receive for breaking a world's record.

Practice of exercises such as are contained in this book, and attention to proper posture will eliminate any condition of flat-chestedness. As you have read in another chapter the bones of the sternum do not become fixed until very late in life. The ribs are constructed in part with flexible cartilages so that they will readily expand. Exercise and proper posture will overcome this condition. First you must have the desire to exhibit a good chest, the willingness to work, and the persistence to continue and to maintain your body in a position of proper posture. You will make gains in

235

leaps and bounds when you continue to strive for a better chest.

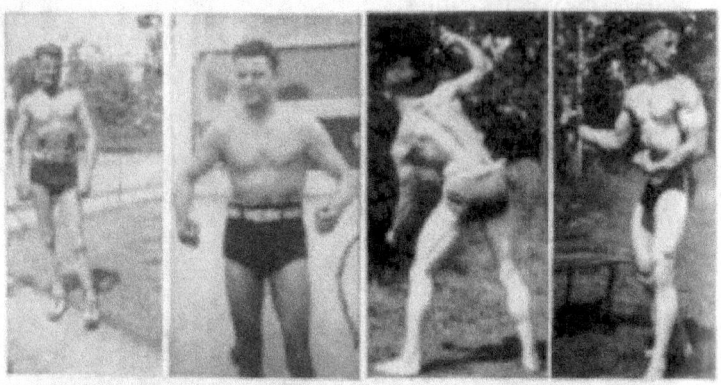

W. P. McDonald, Fullerton, Cal., who gained from 129 to 154 in a year's training time. His chest increased from 36 to 41 inches. He's a business executive.

Ed Koudinski, Minneapolis, Minn., who gained from 116 to 156 in the Great Strength and Health Self-Improvement Contest. His physique improved in a startling manner.

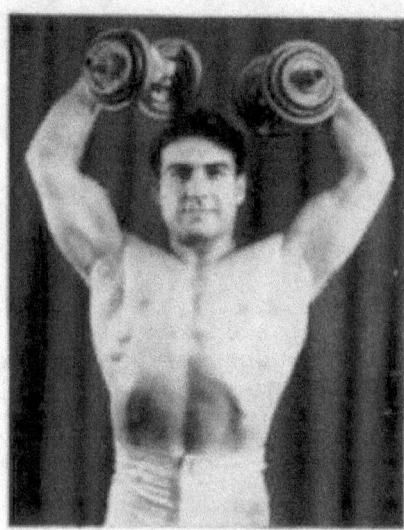

Tony Terlazzo performing one of his favorite dumbbell exercises.

There are definite differences in the chest. My own deeper-than-normal chest, for instance; flared out box-like at the bottom and was comparatively flat at the top. This condition of flatness in the upper chest has been eliminated to some extent but my chest is not as rounded as it might be. This is a natural characteristic which I have been able to overcome only in part. Some men naturally have a round chest and this type of chest with a really fine development of the pectoral muscles is most impressive. The man who has exceptional development of the pectorals, yet walks round-shouldered and flat-chested, is never admired. In fact the very development of the pectorals coupled with his poor posture may lead some to believe that he is subnormal in some respect.

All men will not have the same type of chest for there is so much variation in construction of their skeletal framework. So when you are ambitious to gain a certain type of chest select a model who has somewhat your type of skeletal framework. Men like Grimek who are heavy-boned will obtain a different development than men of the same height who are light-boned. While a short man such as Art Levan, Dick Bachtell or John Terry can attain a forty-inch chest, and a man like Tony Terlazzo, only two inches taller, a forty-four-inch chest, this same forty-four-inch chest might be all that a well-built six footer could hope to attain in his first years of practice. The skeletal framework of some men is so constructed that they have depth first and can more easily obtain width with resulting large measurements and permanent expansion of the rib box.

Posture first; then development of the muscles of the front of the chest, the upper'back and the latissimus, while keeping the waistline as small as possible, will make you known wherever you go as a big-chested man. With constant practice of the chest exercises I have offered, you are sure to obtain a chest which is most impressive in appearance, of more than normal size for your height, one that is a fitting home for sweet-running, powerfully operating heart and lungs.

237

www.ingramcontent.com/pod-product-compliance
Lightning Source LLC
Chambersburg PA
CBHW060245290526
45789CB00001B/194